Dowsing for Good Health

Unravelling the Mystery

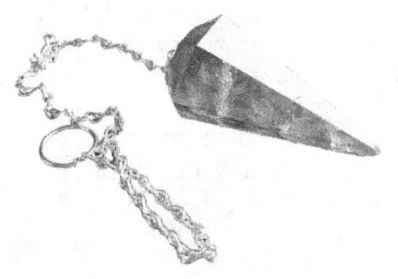

Brenda Hunt

ISBN-13:978-1519144386
ISBN-10:1519144385

Praise for A Beginners Guide to Pendulum Dowsing

This book was easy and reader friendly, an excellent introduction to the world of Pendulum dowsing with a nice little chapter on the history of the topic as well as some of the people that have found their place in history with the use of dowsing.
Having read this from cover to cover I found it to be interesting and full of tips and advice. It has great step by step guidance on a number of different uses including gardening and everyday uses to getting rid of negative energies.
ACLT

A fantastic book for any who want to learn how the use of a Pendulum. Very good history into the Art. Brilliant section on choosing a Pendulum and how to make It work for you.
SP

This book is very well written and is an excellent "starter's" manual for using pendulum. The author includes the history of dowsing, as well as instructions on various methods of using one's pendulum. This book is well written, and the author has a very comfortable and easy style of expression.
I like how clear and informative this book was in getting started with a pendulum. Recommended this book to my family.
Amazon Customer

Introduction

Keeping yourself healthy in the modern world can be a minefield

There is so much information and advice everywhere you turn nowadays, and so much of it conflicts. You can even get conflicting stories in the same newspaper on the same day!

We are surrounded by experts telling us what we should eat, what we shouldn't eat, what we should drink and shouldn't drink, how much exercise we need, what type of vitamins and supplements we should take and - of course - what we shouldn't take!

It's hardly any wonder that most of us end up so confused and also end up ignoring almost anything that comes in the form of expert advice, sometime even giving up on the idea of taking control of our own health at all.

Dowsing is a wonderful way of helping you cut through the all confusion and helping you focus your mind on what matters to you and your family, helping you take back control of your health and your life and finding a path that suits you.

Of course, it goes without saying that you should always consult your doctor if you have a serious illness, and that includes headaches, pain, nausea, fever and any other ailments that persist for more than a few days.

Even if you are taking over-the-counter pain relief, you should seek medical advice if the symptoms last longer than three or four days, or much sooner for a young child or infant.

Working with your dowsing pendulum is a way of clarifying your choices, clearing your mind and finding the best therapies, treatments and answers to help you put your health and your life in balance.

About dowsing

Dowsing has been used by people from the earliest times. It was a tool of ancient civilisations, whether dowsing with rods or sticks or, in more recent centuries, dowsing with a pendulum.

When you first mentioned dowsing to someone, they will automatically think of dowsing with a forked twig for water, and indeed this is a very practical use for the skill of dowsing. Everyone needs water - for themselves, their animals and their crops. Water is absolutely basic to survival and the growth of any community, so obviously the ability to find water is a very valuable skill and the person that has that skill will be valued in their community.

But dowsing is certainly not limited to the search for water.

Dowsing can be used to help you find all sorts of things as well as the answer to many different questions in all of areas of life.

You can dowse to make decisions, you can dowse to find things you have lost, you can dowse to balance energy and of course you can dowse to find a source of water or oil or almost anything else.

I have written a number of books about dowsing if you would like to read further on the subject, but in this particular book I am concentrating on how you can work with your dowsing pendulum to make decisions specifically about your health and well-being.

Although this is not a full introduction to dowsing, if you are completely new to this skill you do need some basic information to help you to get started.

Your image of somebody dowsing may be of a person standing in a field with a forked twig or bent pieces of metal (the rods).

As a child on the West Coast of Ireland, my mother always worked with a forked stick when she was dowsing for new water sources, and many people do like to dowse with the traditional rods, but personally I prefer to dowse with a pendulum as I find it more convenient to carry and easier to work with, especially on the more personal area of dowsing for health.

Basically a dowsing pendulum is a weight at the end of a chain or cord.

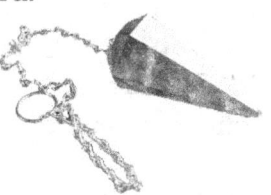

The weight or pendulum will move in different ways to give you different answers. Although you can dowse with a key on a piece of string or a necklace on a chain, it is easier to dowse with a proper, shaped pendulum simply because the weight balance will be more accurate.

You can find dowsing pendulums made of wood, metal, glass or gemstones, and any of them will make a perfectly good tool for dowsing with.

Again personally, as a crystal healer, I prefer to work with a pendulum that is made from a gemstone, a healing crystal, purely because I am more comfortable when working with the energies of crystals.

I have a number of different pendulums and tend to prefer working with either a clear quartz, an amethyst or rose quartz, although I do have quite a collection of other crystal pendulums such as labradorite, carnelian and astrophyllite.

The actual crystal that your pendulum is made of will not have a significant effect on your dowsing. It is just that, as a crystal healer, I feel more tuned into the energy of the crystals and will sometimes choose which pendulum to work with simply because I feel drawn to a specific crystal at that time.

How to dowse.

Once you have picked a dowsing pendulum that you are attracted to, you will need to tune yourself into it.

This is simply a matter of working with it, carrying it around with you and practising until your pendulum reacts easily for you. Once you become used to pendulum dowsing you can pick up almost any pendulum and work with it, you just have to get used to the energy of dowsing in the first place.

Over many years of teaching people how to dowse, I find the best way to become comfortable with dowsing is to work with your pendulum rather than trying to force it to your will.

So although you may have the idea that the 'yes' answer should be a clockwise circle, you might find that for you with a particular pendulum, it is a left-right movement. There isn't a right or wrong way, just the way that is comfortable for both you and your pendulum.

I always find that it is best to get comfortable with a new pendulum.

I always advise students - no matter how comfortable they are with dowsing - to programme any new pendulum before working with it so that they have an accurate match between their own energy and that of the pendulum.

This means that when you do start to work with it for a dowsing session, you are already comfortable with the indicators you will receive from that particular pendulum.

Start your programming session by sitting comfortably in a place where you will feel relaxed and where you won't be disturbed or distracted.

Calm your thoughts and empty your mind of negative energies. This is particularly important when you are programming your first pendulum and are unsure about dowsing. Don't start this process by thinking it won't work. As with anything you do, negative emotions or energies will interfere with any type of energy work and will certainly interfere with the accuracy of pendulum dowsing.

If it helps you to relax, you can play soothing music, use aromatherapy oils or light scented candles, although there are times when you should avoid one or more of these. For instance, you should avoid using aromatherapy when you are trying to find the correct aromatherapy treatment because it might influence your sessions.

Take a deep breath and let it out slowly to calm yourself. Imagine yourself in a bubble of calm energy, for some, it helps to imagine a calming white light or energy surrounding them.

Sit comfortably but do not cross your legs, allow your energy field to be open. You don't want to trap the energy around you.

Hold the pendulum gently between the thumb and forefinger of your dominant hand, letting your wrist relax. You are simply holding the pendulum securely so that it will not fall from your hand, you are not gripping it or moving it yourself.

You are working with a dowsing pendulum, so ask it to work with you.

Ask your pendulum to show you its 'neutral' or 'don't know' indicator.

Normally the pendulum will hang still or will vibrate gently on the end of its chain or cord, but don't force any movement. You are asking the pendulum to show you what indicators it will use, rather than trying to program and force it into your own choice.

You can ask the question out loud or simply in your mind, whichever you are most comfortable with.

Always be polite to your pendulum, you are asking it to work with you, so don't simply demand that it works.

Once you are happy that you know the neutral indicator, ask the pendulum to show you its 'yes' answer and wait for a response.

The pendulum should start to move, often in a clockwise or anticlockwise pattern, but sometimes it will be left to right or backwards and forwards. Be patient, you might not be in tune with the energy of your pendulum straight away and it can take a few sessions before you begin to see a response, each individual is different

Whatever the pendulum shows you is the 'yes' indicator for you with that pendulum.

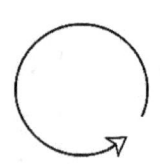 You may find that you have different indicator patterns with different pendulums. My normal patterns are clockwise for 'yes' and anticlockwise for 'no'. But when I work with a carnelian pendulum, I have left to right for 'yes' and forwards and backwards for 'no'.

Ask the pendulum to return to its neutral position.

When it has come to its resting position, repeat the process asking the pendulum to show you its 'no' indicator. This will normally be the opposite of your 'yes' indicator.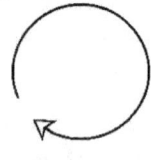

You might find that you can programme your pendulum almost immediately and as you become more practised the process of programming a new pendulum will become automatic.

However, if you are new to dowsing it may take you a few days or even a couple of weeks be for you are really in tune with your pendulum. So don't get despondent, just keep practising until the pendulum begins to react to you with ease.

Advanced programming

As you do more work and more detailed work with your dowsing pendulum, you will probably find that you require more subtlety in your answers.

At this stage you have only asked your pendulum to show you 'yes', 'no' and neutral.

The strength of the answer is reflected in the strength of the movement.

For instance, if your 'yes' indicator is to move clockwise, a small circle will indicate a weak positive while a very large circle will indicate a very strong answer. But there are times when it would be helpful to have more information than this.

Although it is tempting, you shouldn't move onto this stage too quickly. You must be confident in your dowsing ability and in working with your dowsing pendulum before you try to work with more advanced programming, otherwise you will simply confuse the responses, reduce the efficiency of your dowsing and undermine your confidence.

Once you do feel comfortable with your dowsing these are some of the other indicators you can ask it to show you.

A pendulum will not show you these answers until you to ask it.

A 'yes' or 'no, answer to your dowsing can be very helpful, but there are times when a little more clarity would be useful.

'Yes - but' can show you that the general answer to your question is 'yes', but that it's not quite that straightforward.

For instance, if you are asking if apples are a good food for you the answer might be 'yes - but' only if they cooked. Raw apples might cause you problems with acid indigestion.

You might ask if you should add a supplement to your diet and the answer might be 'yes - but' not yet, or 'yes - but' not alone, it needs to be taken as part of a combination of supplements.

In the same way a 'no - but' indicator can also show that the answer isn't straightforward. In either of these cases you would then go on to ask further, detailed questions.

As I said, with most pendulums, my 'yes' indicator is a clockwise circle, my 'yes - but' indicator is a clockwise oval. The same is true of the 'no' indicator, an anticlockwise circle and then an anticlockwise oval. I can also use tell the strength of the 'but' by how squashed the circle becomes. If it is slightly oval there is only a small 'but' in the answer, if it is very oval then there is a very big question mark in the answer.

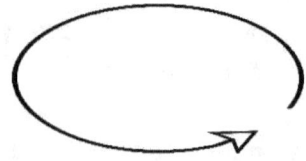

You can also ask your pendulum to show you its indicator for an unanswerable question.

Some questions just don't have a clear 'yes' or 'no' and neutral doesn't really tell you that.

Even the 'yes - but' or 'no - but' sometimes isn't suitable. It's not that there isn't a clear answer, it's more that you've asked question to which there isn't any answer.

You can also call it the stupid answer, because you might be genuinely asking a stupid question. And by stupid, I mean a question where you already know the answer and you are really just using the pendulum as a toy. This is most likely to happen if you are using your pendulum as a joke or as a sort of party trick. If your question is genuine, it is never stupid.

When you get this response, you know that you need to rephrase your question much more carefully, or possibly shouldn't ask that question at all. You should always respect your pendulum dowsing and not allow other people to persuade you to use it as a party trick. If you don't take your dowsing seriously and trust the answers that you receive, you are unlikely to have successful outcomes.

You can also ask the pendulum to show you a 'can't answer' response. This is useful if you have asked a question that literally can't be answered, rather than has a neutral or don't know.

This movement will tell you that there may well be an answer, even a clear answer to your question, but for some reason the pendulum cannot tell you what it is this time.

My own pendulums have diagonal movements for these two responses one diagonally to the left, one to the right.

You probably won't see either of these answers very often except when you ask your pendulum to show them and you will not see them at all until you do programme the pendulum to give you that type of response but they are very useful when you want to be much more detailed in your dowsing work.

Dowsing methods

Once you have become comfortable with your dowsing pendulum, you can begin to work with it in various different ways.

There are basically two methods of dowsing.

In the method you will use most of the time, you are asking questions of your pendulum.

In this case you will be working with the 'yes' and 'no' indicators and any other indicators you have programmed.

But there are also times when you aren't asking specific questions, but you are asking the pendulum to react directly to energy. In this case you do not ask your pendulum to give any particular response, you just ask it to balance the energy and allow it to move as it chooses until it comes to a halt. In this method you are working with your pendulum to rebalance energy and when it returns to the neutral position, that indicates that the energy has been brought back into balance. It is a very useful method when you want to unwind pain or balance the chakra system.

In most of your dowsing sessions will be asking a set of questions of your pendulum as you work your way through to an answer, and this is a general guideline on approaching any such dowsing session.

Try to find a quiet space with calm positive energy, you can play some soothing music or light some scented candles or use aromatherapy to create the right atmosphere for you to work in. You could also prepare for a dowsing session by meditating or do breathing exercises. Imagine yourself in a bubble of calm, positive energy. I often try do take my dowsing outside into the garden, especially on a warm day.

Try to avoid areas of negative energy or strong electromagnetic energy, unless the presence of these energies are part of your question. For instance: -

Can I work in this room if it is full of electrical equipment?

Or is this house to close to electricity pylons?

But in most cases you will be able to control the area for your dowsing session and it is far better to find a place with calm, positive energy.

One of the most important parts of dowsing is to select accurate questions in the first place and it can be very useful to take some time to work out what your questions actually are before you even reach for your pendulum.

Of course, some sessions are more complex than others and will require a set of more detailed questions, while others are very straightforward.

It is very important to be clear in your request for your pendulum. The question has to be phrased in a way that give a positive or negative, the 'yes' or 'no' answer. The question must be clear and precise if you are going to get a useful answer from your dowsing.

This process will also help you avoid the danger of being too casual with your pendulum.

Of course it is perfectly all right to work with your pendulum regularly but it is not a toy. Dowsing should be treated seriously and with respect if you want to be able to achieve accurate answers.

Once you create the habit of thinking about your questions, you will naturally dismiss any flippant ideas and become more serious about your dowsing.

Many dowsing sessions require a series of questions rather than a single question.

For example, if you are dowsing about food intolerance you might simply ask if you should cut bread out of your diet, but this is actually a very wide question and a 'yes' or 'no' answer might not be very helpful.

What type of bread are you asking about?

White, shop bought bread, home-made wholegrain bread, Italian bread with oil, soda bread made without yeast or German rye bread? If you simply ask a broad general question you might get a 'yes' answer, you probably get a 'yes - but' (or 'no' and 'no - but'). But you might only have a problem with the white, shop bought bread that you have in your bread bin at the time. This would mean that you cut all bread out of your diet when you would be perfectly all right with multi-seed breads, Italian ciabatta or Irish soda bread. Even if you have Celiac disease and have to avoid all gluten you can still have wheat free bread

Learning to clarify your thought processes and to be detailed in setting your questions, is a very important part of successful dowsing and a very useful skill to learn for life in general. It helps you think more clearly about everything.

Once you have carefully considered what your questions, are you can begin your dowsing process.

This will vary slightly depending on what type of questions you are putting to the pendulum and I have given more examples of how to proceed with a dowsing session in each chapter.

As you become more confident with your pendulum and your dowsing you will naturally develop your own techniques and your own preferred way of working.

Dowsing with cards

Throughout the rest of this book, I often suggest creating a set of dowsing cards and this is simply a method I have developed over the years when trying to narrow down a list of possibilities.

There are some dowsing sessions that you will repeat quite often, to find answers to different questions from the same set of choices, and in this case it makes it easier to have a set of cards that you can reach for rather than having to take the time to create a list or set of cards each time.

Some people use dowsing charts for the same purpose, where the different choices are written on sections of a pie chart or half circle, but I personally find that individual cards give me more flexibility to add or remove them as I work through a session.

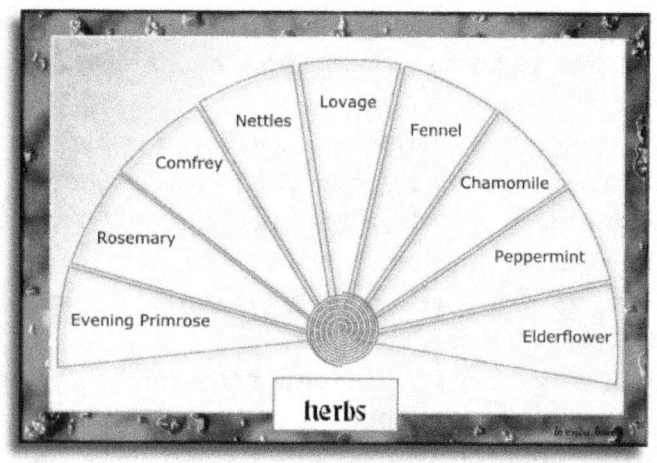

I always advise creating the card set from basic white card, using post cards, index cards or a sheet of card cut into even pieces.

I also write the names with the same pen, avoiding any temptation to individualise them by using colours or adding decoration.

I always use an empty table for the same reason, it's important that your dowsing sessions isn't distorted by any other energies such as a bowl of flowers, a mug of herbal tea or pictures. Without realising it, you could be influenced by the fact that you have some cake on the table when you're dowsing about food choices.

Working with separate cards rather than a single chart, means that you can remove cards from the selection when you receive the 'no' response to the question about that item. It also means that you can make separate piles of 'yes - but' or 'no - but' responses, so that it is easier to return to them as you continue your dowsing session and this will enable you to achieve more detail in your answers.

Finally, it also means that you can arrange your yes answers in order of the strength of the 'yes' response and work with your pendulum to decide which of items you should use now and which in the future, which of them you should combine and other details that will vary with each type of therapy or treatment.

If you are dealing with a very specific question in your dowsing session, one that you will only deal with one time, then you can just use pieces of paper. But there are many areas which you will return to again and again, such as choosing supplements, Bach flower remedies, aromatherapy or homeopathic remedies. I have a set of cards for each of these areas and keep them safely in individual boxes that I can reach for easily, ensuring that I can focus on the purpose of the dowsing session, rather than wasting time and adding frustration by having to spend time either preparing, sorting or even finding the cards before I begin.

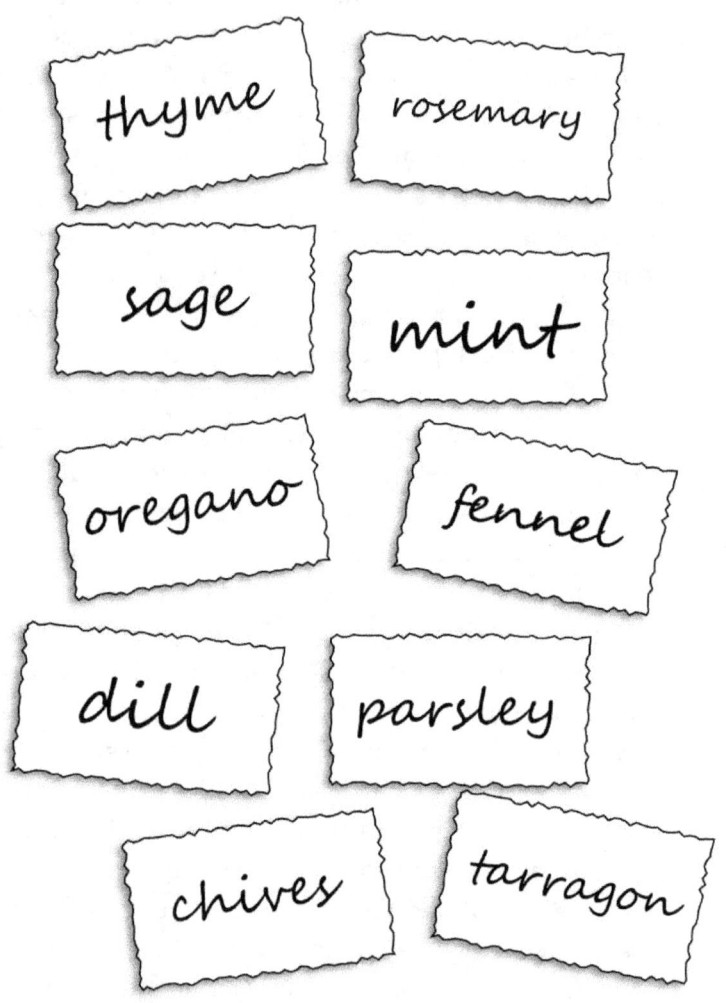

thyme

rosemary

sage

mint

oregano

fennel

dill

parsley

chives

tarragon

Choosing a therapy

You may already have a preferred alternative therapy, in which case feel free to turn straight to the chapter on that therapy.

However, you might be unsure of where you should start in the first place.

Would you prefer working on how to have healthy nutrition and diet, which could also include supplements and vitamins, or do you feel more drawn to energy therapies such as crystal and colour healing and Reiki.

As we have become more in-tune with alternative therapies and complementary medicine over the last few years, the choice has become larger and can be very confusing when you first begin to look at this area of health and well-being. So your first questions might be about which type of therapy to choose.

Of course, there is nothing to stop you using many different therapies.

Although my first love is crystal healing and all areas to do with energy healing, I'm also fascinated by and have trained in nutritional therapy, aromatherapy and herbalism.

I believe that all types of natural medicine can work together to make us healthier, happier and more in balance with ourselves and the earth.

If you are trying to decide on the therapy or therapies that you will work with, you can use your dowsing pendulum at this very first stage of your journey.

As I said in the last chapter, over the years I have developed a process that I call card dowsing for choosing between different alternatives in a dowsing session.

I prepare a set of cards to dowse over.

I like to use index or record cards or plain postcards, but you can cut your own cards from a larger sheet, and the quality of the card or paper will depend on how long lasting you want your set to be. Is it just for a single session, or is it a set that you will protect, look after and return to again and again?

Whatever quality of paper or card you decide to use, all the cards should be the same size and should be plain - preferably white.

Don't choose cards that have any decoration or anything to identify one from another. There shouldn't be anything about the individual card to distract you from the actual dowsing question.

Using the same pen (rather than a range of different coloured pens) write one of the alternative or complimentary therapies on each individual card.

For example, if you are dowsing to help you choose between different therapies, you would have a set of cards each one with a single therapy on it.

- Aromatherapy
- Crystal healing
- Herbalism
- Reflexology
- Nutrition
- Bach Flower remedies
- Reiki
- Reflexology
- Homeopathy
- Colour healing

And of course any other therapies you are considering.

Once you have your cards, you should place them on a clear, empty table.

Don't leave anything else on the table, for instance a vase of flowers, a box of chocolates, a book or a picture. You do not want anything to interfere with or influence the dowsing session. If you had a plant on the table, you might be more drawn to the idea of Bach flower remedies or aromatherapy simply because there is a plant in front of you.

Place your cards equally spaced on the table.

Choose a time when you will be able to relax and concentrate on your dowsing. Don't start to do it five minutes before you have to make a meal for the family or just before everyone will descend on the room to watch the TV. Dowsing should not be rushed, you have to be able to relax and allow your pendulum to work and show you the answers to your questions. You should also avoid a time when you have a raging headache, have suffered all day with hayfever or are feeling deeply distressed and are looking for a treatment for that problem. Although it is always very tempting to want an answer when the problem is at its most severe, the emotional and physical interference will make it very difficult to approach your dowsing in the calm atmosphere and state of mind that is needed for a successful session. Wait until you can relax and calm your mind before you look for the answers you need.

If it helps you to create a relaxing space, light some scented candles, or play some relaxing music.

You should also make sure that you are comfortable.

Wear comfortable clothing rather than being distracted by a tight waistband or clothing that is too hot or too cold.

Sit comfortably, whether that is on a chair or on the floor, but don't cross your legs, you want to keep your energy open rather than enclosing it. Of course the lotus position is fine - that doesn't count as crossing your legs, but make sure it is actually comfortable for you rather than just forcing your limbs into that shape because you think it is more appropriate!

Take a deep breath to calm your energy. You can imagine yourself enclosed in a bubble of pure energy or in a white light.

The method of slow breathing is very useful for creating calm at any time, not just when dowsing.

Breathe in gently through your nose, filling the whole of your lungs, counting slowly from one to five.

Let the breath escaped gradually through your mouth, again counting slowly to five.

Breathe without pausing or holding your breath.

Don't force this process. You might find that you have to work up to the count of five. Start by counting to two or three and work up as you learn to relax.

In our modern world, we have forgotten how to breath properly, rushing this basic process of life as we rush everything else we do, grabbing the oxygen we need in much the same way as we grab a sandwich or a coffee as we walk down the street, rather than taking a little time for the process of actually allowing our bodies to work and gather the fuel that they need.

Ideally, you should slow breath for a few minutes - between three and five - until you feel relaxed and calm.

This process will become easier and more natural as you practice and will also have advantages in life in general, helping you to avoid or manage stress. A few minutes of slow breathing can help at any time of the day and in any situation when you need to regain calm, and it's much more straightforward than interrupting a meeting to do some yoga exercises, although of course breathing exercises are the foundation of yoga.

Deep breathing oxygenates your blood and energises the body, helping rid it of toxins, whereas the shallow breathing that most of us do all the time, doesn't have these benefits and allows toxins to build up in the blood, leading to feelings of mental sluggishness, emotional exhaustion and eventually physical illness. So you can see, slow breathing is one of the first ways of improving your general health and well-being and one of the first benefits of learning to dowse.

Once you feel calm and relaxed you can begin your dowsing session.

At this point you are simply trying to narrow down the choices of therapy that you might work with.

Before you start, decide what timeframe you are asking about.

This is an example of where you have to be clear in your question. If you simply ask, 'is this therapy good for me?' you might get a 'yes' response to all of them.

But you don't really need to know if all of the therapies will be good for you at some point in the next 50 years, you need to know what will be good for you in the immediate future, to help you deal with the problem you are concerned with right now.

You might be looking for an alternative therapy to help you with a specific short-term problem such as a persistent cold or the stress caused by exams.

You might be trying to create a new, healthier lifestyle, making changes that you intend to last a lifetime. Or you may be dealing with a serious or long term chronic illness and be looking for a therapy that will help you deal with one of the specific symptoms of that illness.

And of course you may be asking the question for yourself, or for a loved one or close friend.

Now that you have clarified the nature of your pendulum dowsing session and your questions, you can begin the actual session.

Ask your question as you hold the pendulum over the first card on the table.

If you receive 'no' response you can remove that card from the table and put it into one pile.

If you receive a 'yes' response or a "yes' - but' you can leave it on the table so that you can go back to it for more detailed questioning later, but you can separate them into different piles or areas so that you can remember the difference between the straightforward 'yes' and the 'yes - but' responses.

Move over each card in turn, asking your question. Don't get distracted by going into more detail with a particular card, work though them all first and then go back to make more detailed checks.

At the end of this first part of the session, you will have one set of cards to which you received a 'no' response and these can be set aside for the time being.

You might also have some that received a 'no - but' and you will need to ask further questions about these to clarify the answer.

It might be that the answer is 'no' at the moment but that the therapy should be included at a later stage in your healing.

You will also have cards that gave you either a 'yes' or a 'yes - but' response.

Take the 'yes' response cards first.

Although they all gave you a 'yes', there are probably some that gave you a stronger 'yes' than others.

If you have made a note of the strength of the responses as you were dowsing, you can now place them out on the table in order of that strength. If you didn't make a note, simply place them back on the table and dowse over them again so that you can place them in either ascending or descending order across your table. Remember, a stronger movement from your pendulum indicates a stronger answer.

At this point you can begin to ask more detailed questions.

The therapy that has given you the strongest 'yes' response is the obvious place to start.

You can ask if you should begin this therapy immediately, if you should combine it with some other therapy straightaway or allow some time to use only this therapy at first. How much time should you allow? How many other therapies should you introduce at the same time?

Once you have some answers, you will know what type of questions to ask about the remaining therapies.

Should it be combined with your original choice? Should you introduce it immediately? If not, what timescale should you look at?

The type of questions you will choose to ask and the answers that you need, will depend very much on your individual circumstances and you should use your intuition to create your series of questions for each individual session.

You may decide to split your dowsing over a number of different sessions, gradually working your way through to a precise plan.

If you are already working with alternative therapies, you might find that you are focusing your attention on only one or two different therapies at present and feel that you need to move on to more specific decision-making about those therapies or need to incorporate more into your health plan.

There is no set of rules on how your dowsing should work.

I have always found that it is a very instinctive art and you will become more in tune with your dowsing pendulum and with your own thoughts and opinions as time goes on and you become more confident.

In fact, this can be one of the strong benefits of dowsing, that it helps clarify your own mind and gives you more faith in your own opinions and ideas rather than relying on the guidance of others and the logic of the outside world.

We are bombarded with advice, instructions, reports and scare stories about our health and how to achieve healthy lifestyle, much of it conflicting and much of it involving spending large amounts of money with huge companies and organisations that have their own agenda.

Spending some time with your dowsing pendulum can help you focus on what you need rather than on the latest media story or fad. It can help clarify your mind and allow you to work through what is actually important to you and how to improve your own health in a holistic way, improving you mind and spirit as well as treating your physical needs.

The Chakras

The chakra system is a very important part of many alternative therapies and it is certainly worth understanding what the chakras are and how they affect the entire energy field of the body.

I have written a number of books about the chakra system if you would like more detail, *A Beginner's Guide to the Chakra System* and *Dowsing and the Chakra System,* as well as a series focusing on each individual chakra.

This chapter is simply an introduction and an overview to give you a general idea about working with the chakra system, but it is very complex area and I can only scratch the surface here.

We learn about the chakras from ancient Indian Sanskrit texts.

They tell us of the chakra system, centres of energy in the human body, with seven major points arranged along the line of the spine, from the base of the spine where we sit, to the top of the skull.

The word chakra means wheel or disc, which is a good description and they are generally seen as a Vortex, a spiritual whirlpool, when metaphysical energy enters your own energy field, helping you keep in balance and well at all levels, physical, emotional, spiritual, and mental.

Each chakra is positioned at a major centre of the body, coinciding with the endocrine system and it is believed that the chakras balance and control the flow of subtle energies in the body, which is vital when we take a holistic view of healing and recognise that physical illness often has its source in other areas of our energy field.

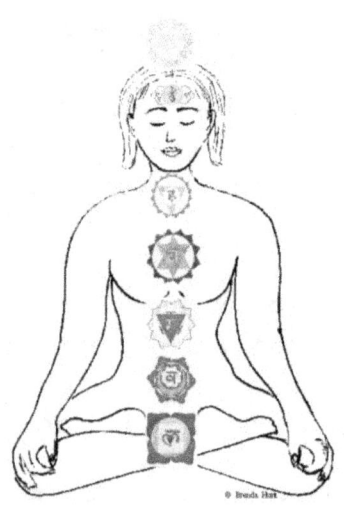

The Root chakra is located at the base of the spine, where your body meets the earth when you sit on the ground. This is the chakra that controls our ability to be grounded. It is associated with physical energy and physical health. If this is blocked you can feel anxious, insecure and frustrated.

Physically it is said to cover osteoarthritis, obesity, problems with the feet and legs, haemorrhoids and constipation and chronic long term illness.

The sacral chakra is located 1 inch below the navel and above the genitals.

This chakra is considered to balance sexuality emotion, desire, creativity, intuition and self-worth.

If it is blocked you may feel emotionally explosive, lacking energy or have feelings of isolation.

Physically it can lead to kidney and uterine disorders, lower back pain, impotence and prostate problems.

The solar plexus chakra is located below the breastbone and behind the stomach. From the back of the body, it is just below the shoulder blades.

This chakra is also known as the power chakra and it is associated with personal power, ambition, anger and joy. It is also considered to be linked to intellectual activity and the central nervous system.

If this chakra is blocked you can lack confidence, worry about the opinions of others, be oversensitive to criticism, suffer low self-esteem or have an addictive personality.

Physically it is said to cover digestive system, stomach ulcers, diabetes, chronic fatigue and allergies.

The heart chakra is located centre of the chest in the heart area.

It is associated with compassion, love and spirituality. When this chakra is out of balance you can feel indecisive, paranoid, fear betrayal or generally feel sorry for yourself.

Physically it can lead to heart disease, asthma, high blood pressure, lung disease and cancers. It is also believed to cover problems with the arms, hands and fingers.

The throat chakra is located just below the collar bone in the throat area of the neck.

It is associated with self-expression, voice, communication and the expression of creativity through speech and writing.

If it is out of balance you can feel that you want to hold back, an inability to express emotions, blocked creativity or perfectionism.

Physically it can cover colds, sore throats, hearing and thyroid problems and tinnitus.

The third eye chakra is located between and just above the eyes. It is associated with intuition, psychic ability, energies of the spirit and the elimination of selfish attitudes. If it is out of balance you may feel afraid of success, non-assertive or the opposite, egotistical.

Physically it can lead to headaches, nightmares, eye problems and poor vision or neurological disturbances.

The Crown chakra is located at the crown just beyond the top of the skull.

This chakra is associated with enlightenment, virtuality, energy and wisdom.

If this chakra is blocked there may be a constant sense of frustration, confusion, depression, obsession and no spark of joy in life.

Physically it can cover a sensitivity to pollutants, epilepsy or chronic exhaustion.

Dowsing works very well with energy, indeed it may well be that the dowsing pendulum reacts to an energy that we cannot see - there are a number of theories as to why dowsing works, but the fact that it does work is far more important than exactly how it works.

This means that working with a dowsing pendulum is an excellent way of helping to balance your chakra system or that of someone else.

If you are unused to working with chakra system, your dowsing pendulum can help you pinpoint the exact position of each chakra.

Clear your mind and calm your thoughts and ask your pendulum to show you the position of the root chakra.

Although you know that the chakra is positioned at the base of the spine - the point that touches the earth ground - you might not feel that you know exactly where to dowse.

You know the general area so you don't need to dowse the whole body or even the whole length of the spine, you just need to hold the pendulum about 4 to 6 inches over the general area and ask your pendulum to show you whether you are at the correct position for the chakra. Just slowly move your pendulum around the general area and it will give you it's 'yes' answer when you are in the correct position.

You can do this over any or indeed all of the chakras.

It can also be a very helpful technique when you want to find position of the chakra points on an animal. Although they also have the seven major chakras in line with the spine, the anatomy of a horse is not exactly the same that of a cat or dog and none of them are exactly the same as you.

When you start working with dowsing chakras, you will almost certainly start on your own system and this requires a different method than when you work on someone else.

When you are cleansing someone else's chakra system you can actually dowse over each chakra, but this is physically very difficult on your own energy system, especially the crown chakra unless you have very long arms!

As with any dowsing, find a calm relaxing area in which to do your dowsing session. You can play soothing music or light aromatherapy scented candles if these help you to create the right atmosphere. Make sure that you are comfortable and will not be disturbed.

Calm your mind, take a deep breath and relax.

As always, the first question you should ask is if it is all right to proceed with this dowsing session at the moment.

There may be times when you get a 'no' response, and this might be because you're too tired, too emotionally drained or that it just isn't an appropriate time to work on the chakra system.

Accept this and put your pendulum away for another time.

If you receive a 'yes' answer (which is normal) ask the pendulum to help you in balancing the chakras.

Hold the pendulum in your dominant hand to the side of your body and hold the palm of your other hand over - but not touching - your root chakra.

In this type of dowsing you are asking your pendulum to balance energy rather than give you a 'yes' or 'no' response.

So in this case, rather than looking for a negative or positive movement, you simply allow your dowsing pendulum to move as it wills until it comes to a natural halt at its neutral position.

This is the method of dowsing that you use when you want to balance energy rather than ask a question. It may take a few seconds for your pendulum to settle in the neutral position if the energy is already in balance, or it can take a few minutes if there is an energy blockage that the pendulum is unwinding.

When you are working on the chakra system for any healing method, you always start at the root chakra and move up through the system ending at the crown chakra to allow energy to move up from the earth through your system.

As you are dowsing over each chakra the pendulum will either remain at its neutral indicator, showing that the chakra is in balance, or it will move. If it does start to move, allow it to move as it wishes, for as long as it wishes. Once it comes back to your neutral position you can move the palm of your hand to rest over the next chakra.

Alternatively, you can focus mentally on each chakra as you balance it, rather than holding your hand physically over the area. This method can be easier if you have mobility problems.

The strength or size of the movement in the pendulum indicates the balance, or imbalance of the chakra. If you have an injury or long-term illness you will find that the relevant chakra will stubbornly slip out of balance on a regular basis.

I have M.E./CFS (chronic fatigue syndrome) and I find that my root and throat chakras are frequently out of balance and need more time to rebalance them than any of the other chakras.

As an alternative method with your dowsing pendulum, you can allow the pendulum to move clockwise to indicate that there is imbalance, left to right while it is removing the negative energy, and then anticlockwise while it recharges the chakra with positive energy. If you want to use this method, you have to program your pendulum to do it in the first place. Simply ask your pendulum to use each of these movements for each purpose.

You can use either method depending on which you are more comfortable with. You can also use them on a single chakra as well as the whole system to help ease the specific pain. For instance, on your throat chakra if you have a sore throat or cold, or on your sacral chakra if you have indigestion or a stomach upset.

However, you should not get into the habit of overworking one area, as this will cause imbalance in the system as a whole, so if you do find that you are balancing a single area frequently to ease a specific problem, you should also give yourself time on a regular basis to balance and cleanse the entire system.

You can also work with your pendulum to help balance the chakra system of someone else, your partner, your children or your pets.

You must always check that is appropriate to work on someone else's chakra system before you begin.

Obviously you should ask their permission, but you also need to check with the higher energies before you do any dowsing. The easiest way to do this is to ask your pendulum if it is appropriate to start any dowsing task.

Relax, hold your pendulum loosely between your thumb and forefinger and clear your mind.

Ask your pendulum if it is all right to start this dowsing session.

As long as you receive a positive answer you can go ahead and start dowsing. If you receive a negative answer it might be that it is inappropriate at this time to work on the chakras, or it might not be appropriate at any time for you to work on balancing this particular person's chakra system.

You can ask further questions of your pendulum to check what the correct answer actually is.

As long as you have received a 'yes' answer, you can then start the chakra balancing system.

Ask the person to lie down comfortably on their back with their hands at their side.

Although this is preferable, it is not always possible and I also find that you can use the same general method while they are sitting comfortably with their hands by their sides.

Before you start the session make sure you are both comfortable and in a calm relaxing atmosphere.

Hold the pendulum approximately 4 to 6 inches above the person you are dowsing.

As always, start at the root chakra and allow the pendulum to move as it wishes.

If it stays in your neutral position the chakra is already balanced.

If it moves in either your 'yes' or 'no' pattern, allow the pendulum to move as it wishes, holding it over the chakra until it settles once again into the neutral position, showing you that the chakra has been rebalanced, then move on to the next chakra.

It may take a little while before the pendulum returns to its neutral position, don't try and force this, you are simply allowing the dowsing to take its own pace. If you feel that your arm is beginning to ache, support your dowsing hand by holding the elbow of that arm in the palm of your other hand.

Continue in this way until you have passed over all the chakras ending at the crown.

If there have been any areas where your dowsing pendulum is taking time to rebalance the chakra, you may find that the blockage at that point is more serious.

I find that my pendulum can show me two different types of imbalance in chakra. If it makes a very large pattern that settles down into small movements and then returns to neutral fairly quickly, it is normally showing me that the person has a strong pain or problem but that it is fairly easy to rebalance, such as headache, a pulled and painful a muscle, or temporary upset in their lives.

On the other hand, if the pendulum makes a steady pattern, maybe not a large dramatic swing but one that takes much longer to settle back to neutral, the imbalance in the chakra is much more deep-rooted and this could indicate a serious medical problem, a deep-seated emotional blockage possibly even carried forward from a past life, or they are dealing with a deep-seated spiritual problem.

Dowsing the chakra system should not be considered as an alternative to medical treatment and if you feel that there is a serious physical or emotional problem you should always advise the person to seek professional medical attention. Unless you are professionally trained in either physical or psychological medicine, you should never try to diagnose yourself or anyone else.

When you have completed a dowsing session for balancing the chakras, either of yourself or someone else - especially if there has been a strong blockage - there can be a feeling of light-headedness or a slight dizziness. This is quite normal and you or the other person should sit quietly for a few minutes and sip a glass of water allowing time for the energy to be absorbed.

You can take the information from a chakra dowsing session into your other types of healing. For instance, if you discover that one area of the chakra system consistently needs rebalancing, you can work with other therapies on that part of the body.

The best type of healing is holistic, taking the mind body and spirit as a whole rather than a collection of separate parts, and taking all therapies as a whole, working with them and combining them as you feel they are needed.

You can look upon the chakra system as a map for the body, giving you information about the health of the whole system on all levels, physical, emotional, mental and spiritual. It is the ideal way to see the energy system and, of course, a person as a whole being.

Food allergies

Allergies have become much more common over recent years and there are many theories as to why this has happened.

It is probably a combination of many causes.

More chemicals in daily life, more central heating, less fresh air, even the increased use of the oils in baby food has contributed to the growth in food allergies.

Whatever the reason, many of us find that we have problems with various ingredients found in daily life and in our food, but it is not always easy to discover what ingredients that you have a problem with or what products the allergen is in.

Although there are specific allergies which can in their most severe form be life-threatening, most of us actually have an intolerance rather than an allergy.

With an allergy our immune system will react against the substance, seeing the food as a threat and releasing chemicals which cause the allergic reaction.

These reactions can be a rash, an itchy sensation inside the mouth or throat, swelling around the face or even vomiting.

In the most serious cases there can be breathing difficulties and light-headedness, this severe allergic reaction is called anaphylaxis and can be life-threatening and indeed fatal if treatment isn't given quickly.

Many people who suffer food allergies also suffer from other conditions such as hay fever, asthma and eczema.

Food allergies are extremely serious and those who suffer from them are normally very aware of the dangers, so much so that they will carry an epipen, an epinephrine autoinjector which is a medical device.

Other people will have an intolerance rather than an allergy to foods.

Although it might not be immediately life threatening, an intolerance can certainly be exceptionally uncomfortable and damaging for your long term health.

An intolerance can cause stomach cramps, bloating and diarrhoea and the symptoms can develop many hours after eating the food. This time delay together with the fact that it is possible to be intolerant to a number of different ingredients can make it difficult to work out which foods are the problem and it is an area where dowsing can be very helpful.

There are two ways to dowse to discover the source of your allergy or intolerance.

You can either line up the actual products that you think you may have a problem with or you can write the names of the products on separate pieces of paper.

You can then either dowse over the products, or the names of the products.

I prefer to use a combination of the two methods.

Initially I will write a selection of potential allergens onto separate cards, in fact I keep a set of cards that I have made so that when I begin working with a new client I already have the set of cards prepared.

Food Allergens

There are quite a number of potential allergens to be found in food products and it is useful to know what they are.

Celery.

This includes celery stalks, leaves, seeds and the root called celeriac. You can find celery in salads, some meat products, soups and stock cubes and core celery salt.

Cereals containing gluten.

The most obvious of this is wheat (which includes spelt and Khorasan wheat) but it also includes barley, rye and oats. Cereals are often found in processed foods which contain flour such as baking powder, batter, breakfast, bread, cakes, couscous, meat products, pasta, pastry, sauces, soups and even fried foods which can be dusted with flour.

Crustaceans.

This can include crabs, lobster, prawns and scampi. Southeast Asian curries or salads can often include shrimp paste.

Eggs.

Avoiding eggs might seem simple but they are often used in cakes, some meat products, mayonnaise, pasta, quiche, sauces and pastries and some foods are glazed or brushed with eggs.

Fish

Although this might seem easy to identify, you can also find fish in relishes, salad dressings, stock cubes and Worcestershire sauce.

Lupin.

You might think of Lupins as beautiful flowers in the garden, but it is also found in flour. Lupin flours and seeds can be used in some types of bread, pastries and even in pasta.

Milk.

Lactose intolerance is a common digestive problem caused by the body having a problem with the type of sugar found in milk - lactose. Milk might be easy enough to identify as a drink but of course it is also found in butter, cheese, cream, milk powders and yoghurt as well as being used in some food that are brushed or glazed with milk. It is also used in powdered form in some soups and sauces.

Molluscs.

These include muscles, squid, whelks and land snails and are often found in oyster sauce or of course as an ingredient in fish stews or pies.

Mustard.

Although it is easy enough to avoid a jar of English mustard, you can also find liquid mustard, mustard powder and mustard seed used in breads, curries, marinades, meat products, salad dressings, sauces and soups.

Nuts.

Although you might first think of peanuts in this category, they aren't actually nuts. This group refers to nuts that grow on trees such as cashew nuts, almond, Brazil nuts and hazelnuts. Nuts can be used in breads, biscuits, crackers, deserts, nut powders which are often used in Asian curries, stirfry dishes, ice cream, marzipan which is almond paste, nut oils and sauces.

Peanuts.

Peanuts are actually part of the legume family and grow underground. They can be found as an ingredient in biscuits, cakes, curries, deserts, sources as well as groundnut oil and peanut flour.

Sesame seeds.

These little tiny seeds, which can be very healthy if you're not allergic to them, can often be found sprinkled on bread, especially burger buns. You can also find breadsticks, hummus, sesame oil and tahini, they are also used in salads.

Soya.

Although this can be a very healthy food and is often used in vegetarian meals, it can also be an allergen. It is normally well labelled but you also need to be aware of edamame beans, miso paste and tofu, it can also be found in desserts, ice cream, meat products, sauces and of course processed vegetarian meals.

Sulphur dioxide.

This ingredient is sometimes referred to as sulphites and is used to dry fruits such as raisins, prunes and dried apricots. It is also found in some meat products, soft drinks, vegetables, wine and beer. You have a higher risk of a reaction to sulphur dioxide if you already suffer from asthma.

As you can see from this rather extensive list of potential allergens, it is much easier to start your dowsing process with a set of cards rather than samples of almost every food in the supermarket.

First of all, prepare a set of 14 cards for yourself, each one with just the headline name of the allergen without any further details.

Once you have narrowed it down from the total potential list, you can then produce a second set of cards, one for each of the potential products that might contain the allergen. Alternatively, at this stage you might prefer to go through your storage cupboard and dowse over each product that might include the allergen.

Once you have created your set of 14 cards you are ready to begin the first stage of the dowsing process.

Choose a time when you can calm your mind and approach the dowsing without emotional interferences.

Don't begin dowsing just after you have been affected by your allergy, the emotions of feeling unwell will interfere with your dowsing session and you will not be able to get accurate answers.

Make sure that you are wearing comfortable clothes, you don't want your energy to be distracted by a tight waistband or feeling too hot or too cold.

Calm your mind. Imagine yourself enclosed in a bubble of clear white light.

You can play relaxing music, although at this stage you should avoid lighting scented candles or using aromatherapy as ingredients can be very surprising, for instance, many candles use soy wax and many aromatherapy carrier oils are nut oils.

Use a clear table. You don't want anything on the table to interfere with your dowsing. For instance, if you leave a box of chocolates on the side of the table, one of the ingredients in the chocolates could be one of your allergens, and that would interfere with accurate dowsing.

Place your cards out on the table with space between each of them. Dowse over each card individually, asking your question.

You can phrase your question in a way that suits you, for instance

Is this ingredient an allergen for me?

Is this ingredient safe for me?

Does this ingredient combine with something else to create an allergen for me?

If you have a combination of problems, for instance some things cause a rash, some a stomach upset, or others cause headaches, you should specify what you are looking for at this particular time.

Does this ingredient cause a digestive problem for me? You should always add to the for me so that you know that the response is related to you rather than other people in general or to one of your children or your partner.

As you dowse over each card you can begin to sort them into separate piles. The ones that have a straightforward 'no' indicator can be set to one side.

The ones with a straightforward 'yes' can also be put to one side, although you should make a note of how strong the response is. I keep a notepad by my side on the floor to make notes as I work. Don't keep it on the table, you don't want anything else to interfere with your dowsing pendulum.

Other cards might give you a 'no - but' or a 'yes' - but' response, and you should make a note of these as well.

An ingredient with a 'no-but' might be a problem if it is used raw but not if it is cooked.

Some food items are quite complex and include a lot of ingredients.

This is quite obvious if you're looking at a processed meal or a recipe that includes a number of different ingredients such as soup. But even something that appears as simple as bread can include a number of different items, any one of which could be causing the problem. The obvious ingredient is wheat flour, but bread also includes milk (lactose), yeast and can also include sugar, salt, oil, olives, cheese, onions, sesame seeds and nuts. If you dowse over a card with the word bread on it, you may get a "yes'-but' response. You will then need to ask more detailed questions to discover if you are allergic to the wheat or gluten in the wheat, the yeast or the lactose. You might not need to cut out bread altogether but you might need to choose yeast free breads such as soda bread, or gluten free bread. It is always worth asking additional questions until you get a clear, unambiguous answer from your dowsing pendulum.

Once you have a selection of some items that are allergen or cause an intolerance, you can begin to ask more specific questions, narrowing down which items or food products are more likely to make you react.

Some items can be found in number of different products. Wheat can seem to be almost universal once you start reading product labels, you can find it in the most diverse range of items. Although you expect to find wheat in bread, biscuits and cakes you will also find wheat flour in processed foods, soups and sauces.

At this stage you can collect a range of items that include an ingredient that is an allergen or causes food intolerance problems for you, and dowse over the individual products to discover if you have to avoid them altogether, use them sparingly or continue to use them as normal.

If you have a serious problem with an ingredient, especially an allergy rather than an intolerance, it is wise to always check a new product before you introduce it into your diet to make sure that it doesn't include any trace of the ingredient.

In this case I would recommend having a sample of the actual product to dowse over or writing the exact brand name and version details on a card. Some brands are available in a variety of products. For instance, some beef drinks are available as powdered or paste versions, and not all versions actually include beef. A number of meat flavoured convenience meals don't contain any meat, your chicken noodle meal might contain soya instead of meat and your beef and onion crisps might actually be vegetarian.

So it is important at this stage of dowsing to ensure that you have the exact name and version of the product written on your card if you can't work with a sample of the actual product.

There are also times when you will work in the opposite way. Rather than having a list of ingredients that you might be allergic to, you could choose to have a list of or samples of foods and dowse over them to find if you are allergic or intolerant to any of them.

This can be a very useful method if you find that you are having problems with your digestive system, with rashes, headaches or generally feeling unwell.

Although you might not have an actual allergic reaction to any ingredient, you may well find that some of the foods you have in your regular diet are actually causing your health problems and that you would feel much better in general if you avoided these foods altogether or kept them for special occasions when you are prepared to put up with the discomfort.

You might also find that some of these foods only cause your problem when you overdose on them, which could mean that you choose never to keep ice cream in your freezer but only ever enjoy it as a special treat when you go out for a meal.

Of course, food isn't the only thing that can cause problems. Our homes and workplaces are full of chemicals nowadays. Food containers, cleaning products, even skin care, soap, shampoo and deodorant can contain a cocktail of chemicals, many of which are also used as weedkiller and pesticides, so you should continue your dowsing to cover all the products you use in your home to see if any of them are affecting you.

I cannot use ordinary soap or body wash, it brings me out in a rash, my husband had a serious problem with a type of laundry powder and my mother suffers from very bad stomach cramps if she uses moisturiser or hand cream with a certain ingredient in the mix, and as a family we are not unusual - many people put up with low level discomfort, lethargy, headaches and skin problems which could be solved easily if they avoided certain products.

If you do have a serious allergy rather than an intolerance, you should always consult your medical practitioner as an allergy can be life-threatening and you must make sure that you are aware of it and make other people aware of it.

I have to finish this chapter with another warning.

Do not get too obsessed with searching for allergies and intolerances.

Although it is always very healthy to avoid the foods that cause your problem it is possible to take this to such an extreme that you end up with a very limited diet, and that because can become psychologically addictive as well is unhealthy from a physical point of view.

A good diet helps you live a healthy, active and emotionally positive life, but food is not the enemy so don't allow yourself to treat it as such.

Food or diet plan

Although you not may not be concerned about food allergies and intolerances, good diet is still a vital part of any health routine.

We trot out the phrase 'you are what you eat' without really thinking about it, but it is absolutely true. You are literally what you eat.

The fuel that you put into your system, directly affects how your body will work. How you feel, how healthy or otherwise you will be can all be affected by your choice of meal. We often put more thought into the fuel that goes into a car than about the fuel we put into ourselves.

The basic outline of any health routine has to include a good diet.

The word diet is basically used in either of two ways.

When someone says they want to change their diet, they are either thinking of a weight loss diet or a healthy eating plan.

Although a weight loss diet can have its place at times, the only real way to be healthy and to control your weight in the long-term is to adopt a healthy eating plan for life.

Instead of thinking of surviving on starvation rations for a few weeks, tightly restricting the foods you eat or the way you combine them, or trying to stick to a low calorie diet for a few months, you should really be thinking of making changes in your diet that will last the rest of your life.

This is the only way to choose a healthy diet rather than being trapped into a circle of yo-yo dieting, constantly losing and regaining weight and damaging your long-term health in process.

When you walk through the supermarket it can seem almost impossible to narrow down the vast choice of foods to a healthy selection.

Although you might have dowsed to discover what foods may give you a problem with food intolerances or actual allergies, it is now important to try and discover what foods you should eat for general good health.

There is so much conflicting advice about this. The newspapers are constantly full of stories about foods that you should or shouldn't eat, the latest list of super foods, and the latest list of foods to avoid. It can be almost impossible to decide what you actually should be eating.

Obviously you can look at different websites and different books to give you guidance about a balanced diet, about the levels of carbohydrates, proteins and fats that you should be consuming, but there comes a point when you have to make the theory real and choose actual foods that will live in your store cupboard and fridge.

This is where you can use your dowsing pendulum to help you make these decisions and narrow down the vast range of choices that face you today in a modern supermarket or foodstore.

This is an area where you will work with your dowsing pendulum on a regular basis.

You can certainly have a full dowsing session at the beginning of creating any new healthy eating, dowsing over the actual foods or the names of foods that regularly live in your store cupboard, in order to see whether they should retain their regular slot.

You can ask different questions depending on what information you need. For instance, you might ask a straightforward question of whether you should continue to eat a certain food regularly. If the answer is 'no', you could then ask it would be all right to eat it on occasion as a treat or if you have to remove it from your diet altogether.

It is worth checking with your dowsing pendulum about all the foods that you consume, because there are times when we have been told that a type of food is very healthy although when you look at the labels it can be full of sugars. For instance, some types of healthy breakfast cereal actually have more sugar in them than a chocolate bar.

You might also think that you are doing you and your family a favour by buying low-fat yoghurts, but again they can be packed full of sugar, so the healthy treat might contain more sugar and additives than a cake.

A good first stage is to dowse to check all the foods on your regular shopping list.

You can do this by either removing the bottle, jar or box from the store cupboard and dowsing with it in front of you or by dowsing over the exact name and make of the food.

As with any dowsing session you should do this when you can calm and relaxed and not affected by intense emotions.

So don't do this when you feel bloated from eating something, unhappy at your weight when you stood on the scales, or have just come out in a rash again. You also shouldn't do this at a time when your children have been causing chaos and you want to see if the additives in the food are the reason for this.

Any of these situations might be the trigger for you to decide to check your food choices, but don't do it at that time. Wait until you can be calm, relaxed and distanced from the problem. You will be able to get a much more accurate response from your dowsing if you remove the emotional turmoil from the process.

When your mind is clear, find a time when you will be able to concentrate and be undisturbed.

Place the product on a clear table or bench. You can also write the exact name and brand of the product on a card and dowse over that if you don't have the item in your store cupboard.

The bench or table should be clear other than for the product, so that other items do not interfere with the dowsing energy. For example, it might have an effect if you have a bowl of sugar close to a box of cereal and you're asking questions about the cereal.

Think clearly about what your actual question is.

Do you want to know if the cereal is good for you, are you asking about the health benefits of it or whether you like the taste of it? Or are you asking if the cereal is good for your children?

Some products that are healthy enough for adults are not really good for children, even though it is children that they are aimed at. Some chocolate bars are sold as containing calcium, but milk chocolate includes milk which contains calcium, that does not turn a high calorie, high sugar chocolate bar into a healthy meal.

When you are doing your dowsing, make a note of the responses.

Is it a large movement for 'yes' or 'no', either of these are fairly clear, or is it a very small movement which can mean 'yes' it's all right but maybe not actually good for you. It could also mean that the food is all right now and again. You can go on to ask these more detailed questions, so you might discover that your favourite full fat chocolate milkshake is all right as a special treat now and again but not every day with your breakfast.

Once you have dowsed all the products in your store cupboard, you will have a list of items that should remain part of your regular shopping as well as some items that can be kept special treats, others that you might only eat when you go out for a meal and some you really should throw away.

Once you have created this master list of your food choices, you should continue to check new foods that you may not have considered including in your store cupboard before.

This is especially useful if you are thinking of making changes to your regular diet, for instance changing white bread for seeded granary bread or rye bread from an Artisan Baker.

Although you are constantly bombarded with advice from the media about the latest superfood, it might not actually suit your lifestyle, so it's worth checking before you go out and invest in a shopping trolley full of foods that might not suit you.

You can also dowse to check about the places you actually buy your food.

Most of us tend to do a lot of shopping now in the big supermarkets but there is also a lot more choice of farm shops, shops stocking organic products and health food shops.

It can be very tempting to think that the apples that you buy from the organic food store will automatically be much healthier for you than the apples you buy from the supermarket.

All things being equal, it's very nice to be able to buy organic, slow grown, locally produced food. But it can also put quite a strain on your family finances, so it is worth checking with your dowsing pendulum which foods you should invest in and which foods you can happily continue to buy at the supermarket or grocery store.

Again, you need dowse about each different item. You could do general question such as should you buy locally produced, organic meat as opposed to supermarket meat? You might decide to dowse about which supermarket you should buy your meat from, or about which types of meat you should choose.

You can also work with your dowsing pendulum to make decisions about whether you should buy a premium brand, a supermarket own brand or discount store brand.

Again the responses will probably vary from product to product, and you might find that you will be better buying a premium brand coffee but you can happily save money by buying a budget label tea.

Dowsing before you make a purchasing decision can save you a lot of money and it's certainly a lot easier than buying a sample of every variety of tea.

You should get into a habit of regularly dowsing for food choices.

Our requirements of food and nutrition change over the seasons, due to illnesses or as we age. The correct diet for a young child is different to that for a teenager or adult, and changes again as we move into retirement.

Our body alters as we grow and our nutritional needs change through the years, so it's wise to check regularly that the diet you have chosen is still the right one for you, it will probably need fine tuning on a regular basis as your life style, activity level, stress level, and general health changes over time.

If you are beginning a process of improving your health and energy in general, you will find that your whole body becomes more finely tuned and food that you ate quite happily at one stage, becomes an irritation to you or you simply lose your taste for it.

I used to take sugar in my coffee, but then I decided to cut refined sugar out of my diet and changed to sweeteners, now I take it unsweetened and find it very unpleasant if I accidently get a cup that have been sweetened. I also used to love ice cream but decided that I should cut down on that and only have it as a treat when out for a meal, but now I much prefer to end a meal with a cup of coffee that any kind of dessert.

Listen to your body as you improve your general health levels and work with your pendulum to make sure that you are instinctively making the right decisions.

Supplements and vitamins

Food supplements, vitamins and minerals are a huge area of modern alternative health care.

It would be impossible to cover everything in one small chapter, there are entire stores dedicated to supplements of various type as well as vitamins and minerals in different combinations, dosages and forms.

It can be a very confusing area. In fact, as you read through some of the catalogues or websites, you end up feeling that you need to be taking everything, which would not only be extremely expensive, it would probably also be counter-productive.

So this is an area of health where dowsing can be a very helpful tool to enable you to narrow down the overwhelming choices into a practical number of products.

You can use the card method of dowsing for supplements by creating a set of cards, one for each of the supplements that you are considering.

You could also dowse over the details in a company's catalogue if you can get one., but make sure that you can focus on the details of a single item, various strengths and combinations are often listed on the same page. If you are finding it difficult to isolate a single variation, either write the exact details on a piece of paper or card, or cut the specific details out of the catalogue and dowse over that.

Before you start your dowsing session, take some time to think carefully about what results you want to achieve by taking additional supplements.

Some of them can be used as general tonics. The multivitamin supplements are a good example of this.

Although many dieticians will say that you can get all of the vitamins and minerals you need from a healthy diet, in fact it is quite difficult to get a healthy diet.

Many of the fruits and vegetables have been force grown, and grown quickly, which doesn't allow the sugars and therefore the goodness to develop.

And much of our food has also been transported long distances. The vitamin content of fresh fruit begins to decay as soon as it is picked, so very often by the time it reaches our plates, it no longer has the required levels of vitamins left in it.

It is also acknowledged that in the northern hemisphere most people are deficient in vitamin D, the sunshine vitamin, simply because we do not spend enough time outside in the sun, which means that our body is unable to produce the vitamin D.

Vitamin D is a vital hormone and deficiency has been linked to depression, pain, inflammatory bowel disease, breast cancer and autoimmune disease. But it is possible, although rare, to have too much vitamin D, which can cause high levels of calcium in the blood and can mean that you lose your appetite, you get sick, you feel tired and confused.

This is a good example of how important it is to check that you are taking the right vitamins, minerals and supplements to help keep you in good health. Simply taking everything isn't actually the answer.

As well as vitamins and minerals, there are other supplements such as coenzymeQ10, which we produce naturally in our bodies, but which we produce less of it as we age.

Nowadays we want to retain a fit and healthy body as long as we can, and age is no longer a restricting factor in our plans, we want to be able to remain fit and healthy well into retirement, so we supplement the products that our body is no longer producing itself.

You also need to focus on whether you are asking your dowsing pendulum about supplements that you should take yourself or for your partner or children. Men and women required different levels of different nutrients, and children have other requirements depending on their age.

The choices can become very confusing.

Once you have a clear idea of the results you are searching for, and some idea of the products you are asking about, you can begin your dowsing session.

As with any dowsing, you should do this when you are calm and can concentrate without being disturbed.

Find a calm, quiet place to carry out your dowsing session.

If it helps you to relax you can play relaxing music or light a scented aromatherapy candle.

If you are dowsing from a catalogue you must ensure that you can focus very clearly on one product at a time. If there is more than one product on a page, focus clearly on the item you are asking about and don't look at the descriptions of the other items on the page.

If you are dowsing from a set of cards that you have created, place them on an empty table and dowse over each one individually, focusing all your attention on that one card as you dowse.

As you work through the different products, some will give you a definite 'no' answer and you can set those to one side.

Others will give you a definite 'yes' and again you can set those to one side for the moment.

Any that give you a 'yes - but' response or even a 'no - but' response can be checked again with a more detailed set of questions.

For instance, one supplement may require a second product to be taken with it to get the most benefit from it. In another case you may be looking at a single vitamin and a 'yes - but' could mean that 'yes' you do require this vitamin but it's already included in the multivitamin you would be taking.

You can also ask a series of questions about the length of time that you should take a product for. Some remedies can be useful for relatively short periods of time, such as zinc with vitamins C, which can help protect you against colds and infections. It can be better to take this supplement in the autumn and winter, the cold season, rather than taking it all year through. It can give you more effective protection in this way.

You can also ask your dowsing pendulum about the dose you should take. Many supplements can be found in very different strengths, from quite minor doses to huge doses and the advice about which dose you should take can also vary greatly depending on what you are reading. Finding the right dose for you is a very important part of getting the maximum benefit from your supplements, it's not simply a case of taking the largest amount possible.

And of course you should work with your pendulum to check where you should actually buy your supplements from. Should you buy them with your weekly shop, in the local chemist shop, from a specialist health food store that have a huge selection of supplements, or online from a specialist supplier.

You will find a huge variety of supplements to choose from and a large range of prices for items that seem to be the same, which can make the process even more confusing. Working with your pendulum can certainly ease the decision making.

You should also repeat your dowsing on a regular basis as your requirements will vary between seasons and with changes in your lifestyle and health.

Your body will need different help during the winter to the summer, but stress can also alter your requirements, and stress can be caused by good events as well as the traditional 'stressful' situations.

Holidays, weddings and exciting new homes can cause as much stress as money problems, arguments and difficult work situations. And although the stress is 'happy stress' your body still needs some support to get you through it in one piece.

Although you shouldn't fall into the trap of reaching for your pendulum constantly, you should probably give yourself to make a thorough session about your supplements at least twice a year.

Bach flower remedies

Bach flower remedies were originally created by Dr Edward Bach in the early 20th century.

They are a series of 38 flower remedies and they are designed to work on the emotional energy field body, changing negative energies into positive. Dr Bach's aim was to help people achieve joy and happiness in life.

The most famous of his remedies is the rescue remedy, which is a blend of five different Bach flower remedies, Impatiens, Star of Bethlehem, Cherry Plum, Rock Rose and Clematis.

The rescue remedy was designed to help people deal with emergencies and crises, when there isn't time to make a proper selection from his full range of 38 remedies. It can be used in all sorts of situations where stress becomes a problem. This can be caused by a driving test, exams, a work overloaded, or it can be something much more intense, for instance helping you to deal with a bad accident, a severe shock or a bereavement.

The rescue remedy is essentially a one stop shop for times of emergency, but in order to make the most of Dr Bach's ideas you will need to be able to work with the individual flower remedies.

Dr Bach separated his 38 flower remedies into seven different groups based on different emotional needs.

Within each group the different remedies are intended for different types of that emotion and, as it was Dr Bach's intention that they been seen in the seven different groups, that is the way I have chosen to list them.

These are the short and somewhat simple descriptions of the Bach flower remedies, to give you a guide to the different energies that they have, but you can find much more detailed information about each one if you intend to work with the remedies as a main part of your healing process.

To help with fear.

Rock Rose helps you deal with acute or extreme fears which can freeze you into inaction or a panic attack.

Mimulus helps when the fear is of something specific such as dogs, spiders, the dark or being alone. It can also help if you tend to suffer from fears such as losing your job or being struck by illness.

Cherry Plum is for those who fear losing control, especially losing control of their thoughts. It can help those who fear suffering a nervous breakdown or feel that they are in danger of doing something they know is bad.

Aspen can help those who suffer from unknown fears and apprehension, where a fear is vague and unexplainable but constant.

Red chestnut is recommended for people who suffer the problem of being overly concerned about the safety of others, especially being anxious about the safety of loved ones and having a tendency to fear and assume the worst.

To help with uncertainty.

Cerato can help you trust your own judgement when having to make decisions.

Scleranthus can help you when you are having difficulty in choosing or in making up your mind, it can also help with mood swings that emotional upset now.

Gentian helps those who are easily discouraged or depressed when things don't go exactly right.

Gorse can help when you feel hopeless, defeated and deeply depressed when something has gone wrong.

Hornbeam can help those who are feeling exhausted without the strength that is needed to get through each day.

Wild oat can help those who feel that they are at a crossroads in life and cannot decide which route to take, what their purposes or even what they want.

To help lack of interest in life.

Clematis is recommended for those who tend to be daydreamers and who withdraw from the real-life into a fantasy world.

Honeysuckle helps those who are unable to let go of the past or past events and ignore present life because of this.

Wild rose can help those who have sunk into apathy and resignation and who lack joy in life, being disinterested in making any changes for the better.

Olive can help with mental and physical exhaustion, helping regain vitality, energy and interest in life.

White chestnut helps those who cannot quiet their minds or turn off the clutter of their unwanted and repetitive thoughts. It can also help those who worry constantly.

Mustard is recommended for those who feel suddenly depressed without any specific reason, the type of deep gloom that arrives suddenly and feels like a dark cloud.

Chestnut Bud can help stop you repeating the same mistakes over and over again, it can help you learn from experience and observation.

To help in loneliness.

Water violet can help those who are shy or possibly too independent and proud, and tend to seclude themselves from others, leading to loneliness.

Impatiens can help those who have a tendency to lack patience and are easily irritated, especially by what they see as the slowness of others.

Heather can help those who do not like their own company and constantly feel the need of companionship and an audience to listen to their own complaints and problems.

To help those who are easily influenced.

Agrimony can help those who hide their fears behind pleasure and happiness and a brave face. It can help you to communicate worries and real feelings rather than hiding them behind humour.

Centaury can help those who have not learned to say no, who can be weak willed and easily exploited and imposed upon.

Walnut can be helpful in times of major life changes, it can help you move forward and is recommended at times of divorce, starting a new career or making any major change in life.

Holly helps when you suffer from negative, angry thoughts such as hatred, jealousy, suspicion, envy or resentment.

To help with despair or despondency.

Larch can help those with low self-esteem or who suffer a feeling of inferiority.

Pine can help those who tend to assume guilt and to constantly apologise and take the blame when things go wrong.

Elm can help those who find themselves overwhelmed and stressed by taking on many responsibilities.

Sweet chestnut can help at times of deep anguish or despair. It is recommended for times of desperation.

Star of Bethlehem is recommended for times of shock and trauma, whether mental or physical, which may have been caused by receiving serious news, the aftermath of an accident or a bereavement.

Willow can help those who are suffering a sense of bitterness and resentment, when adversity or misfortune makes it difficult to see anything positive.

Oak can help at times when you need energy and inner strength to keep going, this can be caused by overwork, being an overachiever and not allowing times of rest and recovery.

Crab Apple can help those who feel a sense of shame or self-disgust, who feel that they need to constantly clean or wash their hands. It is a very cleansing essence and can help you to detox yourself.

Concern over the welfare of others.

Chicory is recommended for those who tend to have a problem with possessiveness and are constantly interfering in the lives of others, trying to improve where they see fault.

Vervain can help rein back the strong views or fanaticism of an idealist, reducing the amount of unnecessary effort that they throw at everything they believe in.

Vine can help someone to respect the views and ideas of other people, rather than trying to dominate the opinions of all around them.

Beech is recommended for those who tend to be critical and intolerant of others, giving an inability to accept people as they are.

Rock water can help those who expect too much of themselves and can be inflexible, with a tendency to self-denial.

As well as being able to choose a single Bach flower remedy you can also use combinations of them.

One of the most popular ways to work with the flower remedies is to create your own Bach flower mix.

You can combine a number of remedies, up to seven in a single personalised mix. Add two drops of each remedy to a small bottle of water and take a few sips from it regularly, at least four times a day, keeping the liquid in your mouth for a few seconds before swallowing.

Unless you are a specialist in Bach flower remedies, it is highly unlikely that you will have the full set of 38 remedies in your house and it can be quite confusing to decide which ones will suit you best in different circumstances, so I have found that it is easiest to create a set of dowsing cards to help you make the right choices about which remedies to use.

You can use plain postcards, record cards or simply cut sheets of card into matching, regular sizes.

The card should be white and without decoration and you create your set of dowsing cards by writing the name of each individual Bach flower remedy on a separate card. Use the same pen to write so that they are all identical apart from the different name of each remedy. This means that there is nothing other than the name of the remedy to affect the dowsing.

Dowsing always works best when you can detach emotionally from the question, so avoid beginning a dowsing session when you're feeling tense, stressed, unhappy, or unwell.

Although it is always tempting to reach for your dowsing pendulum when you want an instant answer, that is not always the best time to start dowsing unless you are very experienced and can block out the effect of the emotions.

Find a calm space to do your dowsing session, where you will be able to spend time without being disturbed.

If it helps you to relax you can play soothing music, if you want to work with scented candles or aromatherapy make sure that you avoid any that match any of the Bach flower remedies, you don't want to be affected subconsciously.

You also want to make sure that you are comfortable and calm while you are doing your dowsing session, so try to wear comfortable clothing.

When you are dowsing about Bach flower remedies is a good idea to start by discovering if you want to work with a single remedy or a combination. Although you can combine a number of remedies, it's probably better to limit yourself to a maximum of six or seven, otherwise you will be confusing the different energies and muddling the effect.

As always, start your dowsing session by asking if it is the right time to proceed with this particular dowsing.

As long as you have received the 'yes' indicator from your pendulum you can continue with session.

Keep the problems that you want to treat clearly in your mind, you need to focus on the purpose that you wish to use the Bach flower remedy for.

It's important to be very focused on any of your questions during a dowsing session, because although you might think that you are asking about the problem for yourself, unless you specifically focus your attention on that, your mind and your subconscious might actually be thinking about treating your partner or one of your children, other family or a friend.

If it helps you, you can write down the question you want to focus on. We are physical beings and there is nothing wrong with having a physical item to focus on to help the concentration.

When dowsing about Bach flower remedies, I always find it helpful to start by asking how many remedies I should be looking for.

You can do this by simply asking the question of your pendulum and then going through the numbers - one, two, three, four et cetera - until your pendulum gives you a clear 'yes'.

Having this number in mind will help you in the rest of the dowsing session.

At this stage you can place your dowsing cards on a clear, otherwise empty table. You can either use the full set of 38 cards, or if you have already decided on one of the seven Bach flower groups you can work with the cards for that group.

Holding your pendulum over each individual card in turn, ask your pendulum to show you whether this is a good remedy for you at the moment or not.

If you receive a 'no' indicator you can remove that card from the table.

If you receive a 'yes' indicator, make a note of the strength of the movement of your pendulum. A larger movement means a stronger answer.

Dowse over all your cards until you have a response to all of the Bach remedies. If you have received a strong 'yes' indicator to one of remedies, obviously this is the one you should be using at that time, but you will probably have received different strength answers to a number of different remedies and you may wish to ask further questions before you make your final selection.

As an example, you might ask if those two or three remedies should be combined together or if you should use one now but a different one in a few days' time.

The exact questions you want to ask will depend on your own circumstances, and as with all dowsing you will find that the more you work with a pendulum the easier it is to form questions and to interpret the results.

Although Bach flower remedies are the most well-known, since Dr Bach developed his famous flower remedies others have followed where he led and you can find other brands and ranges as well, and you can also work with your pendulum to decide if you should work with the original Bach flower remedies or another collection.

You can also develop your own range of flower essences, but that's another story or possibly another book.

Aromatherapy

In aromatherapy we are working with the therapeutic qualities of plants to produce a physical, spiritual, emotional and mental sense of well-being.

This can be through massage with essential oils or through inhalation and other methods.

The essential oils are chosen for their different therapeutic qualities, some are stimulating or refreshing and others are sedative and calming. They have been used since earliest times, aromatherapy was used by healers and priests in ancient Egypt, Persia and China.

Although we fell out of love with all types of natural healing when we were seduced by the products of the big pharmaceutical companies, aromatherapy has never really gone away, and has become more and more popular again in recent years.

The term aromatherapy has been used to sell all sorts of products from bath foam to candles, shampoo and body lotions, even air fresheners and cleaning products.

But these products are often simply using chemical scents rather than genuine, natural plant essences and this has in some ways devalued the idea of aromatherapy.

In aromatherapy we work with the essential oil from a plant, which can be very powerful.

They are concentrated plant extracts and can be so powerful that with a very few exceptions, you must never use them directly onto your skin. They must always be diluted in a safe carrier oil or cream before putting them on your skin.

You can also work with aromatherapy oils in water, as in a steam inhalation bath, a few drops in your bath water or to scent a room.

Aromatherapy is a very effective therapy for helping deal with stress, and as modern life seems designed to create stress, this means that aromatherapy can be more and more central to dealing with problems and improving our health and well-being.

Stress can produce all types of tension including muscular tension, and this means that the heart pumps more, we have aches and pains, we can become extremely tired, even exhausted because valuable energy is being burned up dealing with the tension caused by stress.

In the short term this makes us tired, irritable, less effective and less able to find joy in life. In the longer term it can lead to depression and reduce our resistance to infection and disease.

Although many of the holistic therapies can help you deal with stress, aromatherapy can instantly connect you to the natural energies of life through plants.

You can work with your dowsing pendulum in a number of ways with aromatherapy to clarify your mind and help you choose which of the many oils would be best for certain times, problems or situations.

The first stage in beginning any treatment with aromatherapy is to choose the oils you will work with.

Unless you are an aromatherapist, you are very unlikely to have a comprehensive collection of oils in your home to dowse over. Therefore, the easiest way to undertake your dowsing session is to create a set of dowsing cards specifically for asking questions about aromatherapy.

Create your cards using plain white card, I often use postcards or index cards or you can use sheets of white card cut to smaller sizes. Whichever you choose, all the cards should be the same size, they should be white, and they should be plain and undecorated. The only thing to differentiate one card from another should be the name of the aromatherapy oil that you write one to a card, so resist the temptation to decorate the individual cards with drawings of the plant.

Once you have your set of cards, keep them somewhere safe because they are an invaluable tool for any dowsing regarding your aromatherapy.

You do not always have to use the full set, you may already have narrowed your choice to four or five, or even two or three oils in which case you would simply use those relevant dowsing cards.

Once you have chosen the cards you will be using, place them on a clear table. You shouldn't have anything else on the table as this could influence your dowsing, for instance if you have a bowl of flowers, the display may include the origins of some of your aromatherapy oils such as rose or lavender, and this could influence your dowsing.

As always, you should create a calm, relaxing space for your dowsing session. You can still play relaxing music if it helps but you should avoid using scented or aromatherapy candles or oil burners in this particular case, again so that you don't influence your dowsing.

Relax and clear your mind.

Imagine yourself in a bubble of pure white light.

Form your question clearly before you start dowsing.

Why do you want to use aromatherapy oils in this case, what end do you wish to achieve?

Are you dealing with something relatively short term or a problem that is more deeply ingrained? You must focus clearly on the purpose of your dowsing.

First of all, ask your pendulum if it is all right to continue with this dowsing session.

As long as you receive the 'yes' indicator you can continue.

If you receive the 'no' indicator you could ask further questions to try and discover why you are receiving the 'no'. It could be that it is the wrong time to ask this question, it might be that you are too emotionally involved at that point to ask the question. If you do receive the 'no' indicator and you cannot clarify why that is, you should put your pendulum away for the time being and come back to it at a later stage.

You should never attempt a dowsing session when you are too emotionally involved in the problem. For instance, don't reach for your pendulum when your back is really hurting and has been giving you pain all day and you are now so tense and so stressed that you will not be able to get a clear answer from a dowsing session.

As long as you have received the 'yes' indicator you can start dowsing over each different card in turn.

Keep your question clearly focused in your mind as you dowse, don't allow your mind to wander as this will affect the accuracy.

If you receive a 'no' indicator over a card you can put it to one side, if you receive a 'yes' indicator, make a note of the strength of the answer. The bigger the movement of your pendulum the stronger the 'yes'.

If you receive a 'yes - but' you can ask further questions. Does it mean 'yes - but' not as the first choice at this time and it should be kept for a later date.

Does it mean 'yes - but' it needs to be combined with another oil, in which case you can ask questions about which oils you should use together.

Continue on until you have covered all the different dowsing cards on the table.

You might then want to go back and ask more specific questions or to dowse for more detail about the oils that you received the 'yes' indicator for.

At this stage you might want to clarify how you would use each oil.

Some will probably be used for massage and you will create your perfect recipe with a massage carrier oil such as almond, olive or grapeseed oil and you may need to make up a recipe of a number of different oils to be most effective. Remember you should never apply aromatherapy oil direct to your skin it is far too strong and must be diluted in a carrier oil or cream, otherwise you can cause skin irritation. Of course you can also work with your pendulum to choose which type of carrier oil is best for you.

Once you have created your custom aromatherapy product you can use it to massage on the skin, as a rub to ease pain or to relax you to help ease sleep.

But making massage oil is not the only way you can work with aromatherapy oils.

You can put a few drops into your bath water, you can put a few drops into a bowl of hot water and use it as a steam inhalation or as a foot bath.

You can also put a few drops into water in an oil burner or use a diffuser to infuse your room with the essence and energy of the aromatherapy oil.

Aromatherapy can become central to your life and infusing your home with genuine aromatherapy, chosen and created for their healing energies is much better than simply buying scented home products that might give you a pleasant scent but without any of the healing energy.

You should also take the time to undertake a dowsing session to help you create an ideal mix to help you relax and create a calm atmosphere for your other dowsing sessions.

We all love to have a beautiful scent in our homes and at work if we can control that environment, carefully choosing your own aromatherapy remedies can help create a much healthier and well balanced energy field as well as a beautiful scent.

Herbal remedies

Herbs have been used throughout history and throughout all different civilisations as a source of food, to make clothing and fibres, to make dies for the fibres, to scent living areas, as part of funeral rituals and of course for their healing benefits.

There is a long history of herbal medicine, built up over time as ancient peoples learnt which plants could be used to heal different illnesses and we can benefit today from the vast amount of knowledge that has been collected over thousands of years.

Ancient records tell us of the herbal remedies used by the Romans, the Greeks, the Chinese, Native Americans and in India and we are still able to tap into the wonderful healing benefits of herbs to this day.

Herbal medicine has a very long history. Medicinal plants have been crucial to the health and well-being of mankind from the earliest times. Everything we get, is in some way from the earth, whether it has gone through many chemical processes in our modern world or whether it is in its natural form, grown and nurtured by the soil, the water and sun.

Unfortunately, over more recent centuries the knowledge of herbalism has been looked down upon or even denounced as witchcraft, so that in our modern world many of us have lost any connection with the wonderful and fascinating medicine cabinet provided for us by Mother Nature. But the fact is that herbal remedies can be incredibly powerful and many of our modern medicines are based on them.

Today for most people, their understanding of herbs is as ingredients in recipes or garnishes on plates, or possibly as an alternative to tea or coffee for a hot drink, and they are often dried and crushed into teabags or spice jars so that any goodness has been drained and pummelled out of them before they reach the kitchen.

When we do think of using herbs as medicine we tend to reach for conveniently pill-shaped supplements.

This can give us a very limited version of the healing properties of herbs, but herbal medicine and growing your own healing herbs in the garden or on a windowsill is an easy way to introduce herbal medicine into your world. Simply making your own camomile tea to help you relax and sleep, or a peppermint tea to heal ease digestive problems may seem very simple but, good sleep and ridding yourself of acid problems can make a huge difference to your health.

Working with your dowsing pendulum can help you in all sorts of ways if you want to introduce herbal healing into your life.

You can dowse to find which herbal remedy you should use, in what form you should use it - as a supplement, as fresh herbs, as an herbal tea - and you can dowse about creating your very own herb garden.

Herbs can be introduced into your life in many ways. They can be used to scent your home in a similar way to aromatherapy, can be used in pill form along with your vitamins and minerals and of course they can also be added to your food, improving the taste of your cooking at the same time as improving your health.

The number of herbs and herbal remedies can be quite surprising at first, there's certainly more choice than parsley, sage, rosemary and thyme.

This is an ideal area for creating a set of dowsing cards because you can work with herbs in so many ways and you will find that you will reach for your pendulum on a regular basis once you start to work with them

When you start your dowsing session it is important to be clear about the purpose of your questions.

You might be trying to find which herb you should use for a particular problem, in which case you must keep that purpose clearly in mind.

As well as deciding on what herb you want to use, you will also need to find out what form you should use it in. A simple herbal supplement, smudging with sage, herbs as scent, either fresh or as potpourri, ingesting your herbs as food or an herbal tea.

Your dowsing session may take a while,

You will probably work with different herbs, in different ways, for different purposes and as you become more comfortable with them, they will begin to infuse your whole life.

As always, you should prepare yourself for your dowsing session, ensuring that you are calm and focused.

Place your dowsing cards on a clear table.

You can play soothing music, but if you want to work with aromatherapy or scented candles, make sure that you are not introducing herbal energies into your dowsing area.

Ask if you can begin your downing session. You will normally receive the 'yes' indicator, but if you receive the 'no' indicator you can ask further questions to establish a reason and you may have to put your pendulum away until a later time.

Herbs can be combined, so you will possibly receive the 'yes' indicator to a number of different herbs, some will be stronger movements that others.

You can also dowse to discover which should be the main ingredient in your recipe for herbal healing and which should be added as smaller additions.

And of course you will dowse to discover how you should work with the herbs for that particular healing requirement.

Healing herbs can be used in so many ways that this is an area where you can frequently return to your card set whether looking for a healing herb or trying to decide which herb will suit your new recipe.

As you become more comfortable with working with herbs, you will almost certainly want to be able to use fresh herbs, picked straight from the plant and used in your home. Anyone can grow herbs. Even if you don't have any outside space, you can still have a special selection of your favourite herbs in pots on the windowsill, ideally placed for adding to your soups, stews and other cooking, to add their healthy properties as well as their wonderful taste. And as an added bonus, adding herbs to your cooking will help you cut down on salt as you won't need to add so much for flavouring.

But if you are lucky enough to have some outside space, even if it is just a balcony or yard, you can design your own herb garden.

You can work with your dowsing pendulum to help you plan that garden. Which herbs should you grow? Which variety of that herb? Mint is not just mint - I have eight different varieties in my mint bed and the same is true for many herbs.

If you have more space for your herb garden, you can dowse to decide where in the garden is the best place for your herb garden. Should you keep them all in one formal area like an Elizabethan Knot garden? Should you spread them out amount your borders? After all, they are beautiful plants and fit well in a decorative border - but do take care - you need to know exactly which plants you are picking for your soup, some garden flowers are deadly poisons and you should never risk confusing them with your herbs.

You can dowse actually in the garden if you are laying out a new herb garden. You can work with your dowsing pendulum to find the right part of the garden to plant your herbs, choosing an area that they will be happy in. Happy plants grow much more successfully, so choosing the right soil conditions, the right sun or shade and the right aspect for them is very important.

On a practical level, choosing the right part of the garden is important as well, your herb garden needs to be convenient, easy to look after and easily positioned so that you will actually go out and pick the herbs on a regular basis. So it probably shouldn't be right at the end of a long garden where you will get soaked or cold if you want some thyme to add to your soup, or a bunch of fresh lavender to put by the bedside in your guest bedroom.

Homeopathy

Homeopathy is another very popular form of alternative therapy.

It was developed in the 1800s into a usable system of medicine by Dr Samuel Hahnemann, a German scientist and physician, although it can be traced back to the writings of Hippocrates at least 2000 years ago.

Homeopathy is based on the idea that you can be treated with the substance which would create the symptoms of your problem in a healthy person.

This can make it a little more complicated to find the right remedy than if you are working with aromatherapy, Bach flower remedies, herbalism or any of the other types of alternative therapy.

Whereas something like Bach flower remedies works on your emotions, and the effects of aromatherapy or herbalism are quite direct - if you have a headache you can reach for eucalyptus, lavender or peppermint oils, a ginger or camomile tea - homeopathy takes a little more working out.

You cannot simply reach for the remedy that will treat headaches, because the choice of remedy depends very much on your headache.

It depends on your symptoms and it has to be matched to the exact symptoms and causes of your headache. What brings it on, what type of pain, where the pain occurs, if there are outside influences that aggravate your headache, what makes it worse and any other symptoms that you experience at the same time. As you can see, this can make it quite a complicated process to pick the correct remedy, and dowsing can help with this.

Homeopathy is an extremely safe form of therapy. Although the ingredients can be quite startling, such as mercury and animal venoms, the dilutions are so extreme that homeopathic remedies are totally safe, even for very young children and babies and of course you can also use homeopathic remedies for your animals.

Homeopathy is also limited to a single remedy at a time. It doesn't matter how many symptoms you have, once you put them all into the mix, a single remedy will be the one that you will take.

Because of the extreme dilation of homeopathic remedies, they do not poison, they don't interact with other medications or forms of alternative therapy and they are not addictive.

It can be effective for both acute and chronic problems. Which means that you can use it to treat things like headaches, hay-fever or cold, but you can also use homeopathy to treat long term chronic problems such as arthritis, respiratory problems and digestive problems.

They are also not limited to physical problems.

There are homeopathic remedies that can be used to help with mental or emotional problems such as depression, panic attacks or lack of confidence.

Although it is quite normal for official bodies and government backed reports to dismiss any type of alternative therapy in favour of modern Western medicine, there are in fact the beginnings of a change in the official position. In 2009 the Swiss government undertook an exhaustive review of homeopathy and came to the conclusion that it is indeed effective, which makes a nice change to hear!

There are a huge number of homeopathic remedies and they can be taken in different potencies.

This means that homeopathy can be a little more difficult to understand and use at home than some other treatments. The fact that there are so many different remedies and that you are treating the symptoms rather than the ailment, can make it much more difficult to narrow it down to the remedy that you actually require.

There are 30 or so commonly used remedies and there are books and websites which can help you narrow down the remedy you require by typing your symptoms into a questionnaire.

If you are treating something very complex or you are very new to homeopathy you may want to consult a homeopath in the first instance, but once you have narrowed down the type of remedy you think you might need, dowsing can help you to focus on which remedy you should use, what dose you need and how you should take it.

Homeopathy is available in different potencies, but as a general guide the 30C potency is normally advised for self-help and is the potency that is most commonly available in shops and chemists.

Again as a general guide, a 30C dose would be taken once every two hours for up to 6 doses for something acute and possibly three times a day for less acute problems. You would repeat the dose for up to 7 days and it is best to take one homeopathic medicine at the time rather than mixing them, as you can do with other therapies such as aromatherapy or herbal medicine.

Once you have narrowed down the huge choices of homeopathy to a manageable number, you can create a set of dowsing cards for homeopathic remedies.

As with any of your sets of dowsing cards, use plain, white, same sized cards as your base. These can be postcards, filing cards or a larger piece of white card cut down to a number of similar size pieces.

Write the name of one homeopathic remedy on each card and do not decorate or otherwise individualise the cards, they should all be the same.

Before you start your dowsing session, ensure that you are calm and relaxed and not emotionally involved in the problem you are asking about. Obviously you will have some emotional attachments to the problem, but try not to do your dowsing in the midst of a severe headache, hayfever attack or any other ailment you might wish to treat. The intense emotional involvement will affect your dowsing session and lower the accuracy of it.

As always, before starting any dowsing session you should ask your pendulum if it is all right to go ahead with this particular line of questioning.

In most cases you will receive the 'yes' indicator and you can continue with a dowsing session. If you receive the 'no' indicator you could ask further questions to try and identify why, but it may be because you are too tired, too emotionally involved or too stressed, and you should put your dowsing pendulum away and leave the session until another time when you are feeling calmer and more relaxed.

As long as you have received the 'yes' indicator you can continue with your dowsing session.

Sit comfortably and relax.

You can play relaxing music or light an aromatherapy candle if you find that this helps you to create a bubble of calm.

Place your dowsing cards on a clear table. The table should not contain anything else that might distract your dowsing. For instance, a bowl of flowers, an ornament or a picture might add other influences into your dowsing.

Whereas in some dowsing sessions you may get more than one strong positive result, in homeopathy it is generally advised that you use one remedy at a time to deal with a number of different symptoms, all of which will influence the remedy you choose. This means that for your dowsing you should only receive the 'yes' answer for one of your homeopathic dowsing cards.

Once you have found the correct homeopathic remedy you can go on to check what strengths of potency you should use and how many doses you should take in a day. You can also check how many days you should use this remedy for.

Homeopathic medicine is accepted to have no side-effects and no interactions with other treatments because the remedies are used in such extremely diluted forms. This means that it can safely be used for anyone, including during pregnancy, for very young children and infants and for animals.

However, as with a number types of energy healing it is possible that symptoms will worsen before they improve. This is sometimes called a healing crisis but the effects should be short lived, in which case there is nothing to worry about. If it does continue you can dowse to see if this is alright or if you should stop the treatment and choose an alternative.

In some cases, you can see an improvement almost immediately, for chronic cases you should at least feel a little better within about a week.

As a general guide, if there is no improvement after two weeks then you probably need to use a different homeopathic remedy.

As with all alternative and complementary therapies, you should never ignore symptoms or pain.

Pain is the body's way of telling you that there is something wrong and if a pain or a fever persists it could be a sign of an underlying serious problem and you should always consult a professional medical practitioner.

Although homeopathy can be used as a self-treatment, it is a very complex system and you may prefer to work with a homeopath, at least at first or if you are dealing with a chronic or long term problem.

You can work with your dowsing pendulum to help you find the right homeopath for you.

When you are deciding to work with anyone - whether you are choosing a new hairdresser or a therapist - it is important to be comfortable with the energy of the person as well as finding someone who is professional and well recommended, but it is especially important when you are looking for an alternative therapist as the energy balance is vital in healing.

There are a number of things that will affect your choice of homeopath, and the individual requirements will differ with your circumstances. For instance, you might be prepared to travel very long distances to work with someone who specialises in a specific chronic illness, but that would be difficult to do on a regular basis.

You will also have your own idea of what it local and what is long distance. Some people commute 100 miles to work, while others feel that a 10-mile trip is a long journey for them.

Taking all this into account, make a list of the homeopaths that are available to you and dowse over their names, keeping in mind the reason for you choosing a homeopath. You may only need a single visit, in which case you can travel further, or you might want to work with the homeopath on a regular basis, in which case convenience has to be considered as well.

Think carefully about what you are looking for and who the consultation if for - yourself, your partner or a child - and prepare your questions before you begin your dowsing, but be prepared to adapt and ask new questions in response to the answers you receive.

It is worth spending time to select the right therapist so that you find someone who is not only a good homeopath, but someone you will be comfortable in working with.

Choosing your exercise

Exercise can be a very thorny issue.

What is exercise?

To some people, exercise is a matter of spending hours in the gym, lifting weights, running on a treadmill and doing miles on a bicycle that never moves.

To other people exercise is moving from the sofa to the kitchen to get another packet of crisps.

Obviously most of us have a happy medium.

At its most basic, exercise is the process of moving your body.

It can help you stay fit, lose weight, reshape your body, keep your mind active, improve your emotional state and improve your metabolism. In other words, exercise is good for you.

We were not designed to be sedentary. We were designed to be on the move constantly, to be chasing our food, working in the fields and walking miles a day. And although we might not have that hunter gatherer lifestyle any more, bodies haven't changed that much and we do need to move them more than most of us manage.

So adding exercise and making sure that you are having the right exercise is a very important part of being healthy.

The thing is, there are so many different types of exercise and so much written about exercise.

The stores are full of books and DVDs, the newspapers and magazines are full of stories and even on the TV we are constantly bombarded with exercise plans and adverts for exercise equipment, and you can spend all day sitting in front of the computer reading about exercise - but that doesn't do anything to improve your health and fitness.

It can get so confusing that you end up doing no exercise at all.

Choosing the right type, the right amounts and the right time for your exercise can be quite confusing.

It's all too easy to sign up for a gym membership, especially on 1st January, and then never visit again which will leave you feeling guilty and out of pocket, neither of which help improve your health or lower your stress levels.

So invest some time in finding what is right for you.

Before you start your dowsing session you should think seriously about the types of activity and exercise that would suit you and your lifestyle.

There is no need to dowse over the entire spectrum available nowadays, it will be quite obvious that some types of exercise simply will not suit you or your lifestyle.

After all, it would be difficult to decide to trek to the North Pole or climb Everest if you have young children to look after at home, although it's not unheard of.

But don't dismiss anything totally out of hand.

I thought I wasn't at all interested in swimming. Couldn't see the point of getting cold and wet for fun, I do live in the north-east of England!

But a friend practically dragged me along to swimming lessons years ago and I discovered that actually, I love swimming and it's one of my favourite forms of exercise, one which I find very relaxing.

So keep an open mind.

You can either create a set of dowsing cards for different types of exercise or you can just prepare a list and concentrate on each one individually, asking your pendulum whether this is a form of exercise you should choose.

The second method is the type I prefer for this type of dowsing, but it's entirely up to you, you should always choose the method you feel comfortable with.

Making a list is a very important part of this type of dowsing where you are choosing between different options. If you don't make a list, you will miss some things out.

You don't have to list every type of exercise that exists, Ironman competitions might be completely out of the question for you.

But do try to be inclusive.

You don't just have to train to run a marathon, taking a walk every day is exercise. In fact, any movement that you don't do the moment is exercise, it will mean that you move more and burn more calories than you are doing now, which is exercise.

So doing the gardening, taking the dog for a walk instead of getting someone else to do it, doing the ironing instead of paying a service or riding a bike instead of taking a car or public transport, all of them are forms of exercise.

So put them on your list with swimming, going to the gym, using the rowing machine and joining a Pilates class.

Once you have your list - and it may take you a few days to feel that you have a right selection for you to consider - settle yourself and start your dowsing session.

As always, you need to be calm and not too emotionally swamped to be able to get accurate answers from your pendulum.

Don't try to dowse when you're upset, when you've just stood on the scales and discovered you gained a few pounds or when you've just tried on your favourite special outfit and found that it doesn't fit as well as it did. And certainly don't reach for your pendulum if someone has just made an unkind comment about your fitness or figure.

Make sure that you are calm and relaxed.

Find a place and time where you will be undisturbed. Turn your phone and emails off, the outside world can wait for a while.

You can play some relaxing music and light candles or use aromatherapy if it helps you to create the right atmosphere for your dowsing.

Wear comfortable clothing and settle yourself so that you can relax and focus.

You might want to place a notebook beside you so that you can make comments as you go to remind yourself of the answers you get from your dowsing pendulum.

As well as preparing your list of potential exercise choices, you should also prepare your questions. You need to know what you are asking about. Why do you want to exercise?

Ideally you should be exercising to improve your overall health. Obviously that will include your physical health, but the right exercise can improve your emotional, mental and spiritual health as well, and exercise should become part of your lifestyle. But there will be times when you have a short term goal in mind for your rush to exercise.

You might want to drop a few pounds for a holiday or special event, you may need to recover from an injury or illness or to train for a charity event.

All of these things will have an effect on your dowsing session and the type of exercise will be suitable for you, so it's important to be clear about your present goal and the timescale if you want to get accurate answers.

Take a deep, relaxing breath and imagine yourself in a bubble of calm energy.

Ask your pendulum if it is the right time to begin this session and to ask your questions.

You will almost always get your 'yes' indicator to this question. If you get the 'no' indicator, you can ask some further questions to find out why, but it will probably be because you are too tense, too emotional or possibly not approaching the question seriously. You should always respect the dowsing process and never treat your dowsing or the pendulum as a toy for a party trick.

As long as you have received the 'yes' indicator you can proceed with your dowsing session, holding your purpose for exercise firmly in your mind throughout.

Looking at your list, concentrate on the first type of activity and ask if this is the method of exercise you should choose at this time for your purpose.

If you receive a 'no' response you can cross it off your list, if you receive a 'yes' you should make a note, you will go back to them later for more detail. At this stage you just want to narrow your choices.

You might also get a 'yes - but' or 'no - but' indicator for some type of exercise and this will mean that you have to ask further questions to clarify the answer. 'yes - but' not at this time?

Should you add this type of exercise into your regime in a few months?

Or should you do it now, but just for a few weeks and then move on to a new exercise as your strength increases?

Equally with the 'no - but' response, is it a type of exercise that you should take up in the future?

Should you think about it again once your injury has healed or once your fitness has improved?

Once you have dowsed through your original list, you will probably have a list of 'yes' responses rather than a single one, and you can now focus on this new list to get more detail for your plan.

For instance, you may have received the 'yes' indicator against your question about using the gym. Now you need to know what type of use you should make of the gym.

How often should you go?

How long should your sessions be?

Should you join a class?

What type of class?

You might have a list of classes offered at your local gym and at this stage you could dowse through them.

Yoga? Pilates? Zumba? Beginner sessions or intermediate standards? Morning, afternoon or evening? Or should you just use the exercise equipment?

And again, which choices would be the best for you at this time and for how long?

Success, or more importantly failure, depends on making the right choices. If you join a class instead of working on your own you might love or hate it depending on your personality and the people around you. You might prefer the company of others, or a chance for some personal time. If you make the wrong choice you might simply give up going to the gym altogether.

Drilling down to the detail that will suit you can be used any type of exercise.

Should you choose running, jogging or walking?

If you choose walking should it be a 15-minute walk twice a day that you can slot into your existing timetable or a long hike or ramble at the weekend?

You could choose to do the 1000 miles a year challenge, but it's up to you whether you do a 20 mile walk each weekend or 3 miles every day.

When you work with your dowsing pendulum you can make decisions and choices that will suit you, your fitness levels and your lifestyle.

As you travel on your exercise and fitness journey, you should repeat your dowsing session on a regular basis so you can check how you should adapt your exercise choices as your fitness levels change.

Life constantly moves on and so should your choices and habits to keep them relevant to you and your lifestyle.

One of the most important thing to remember about any activity is that you should enjoy it. If it's fun, it won't feel like exercise, it won't be a chore that you dread and try to avoid. It will be something that you look forward to, do regularly and get benefits from.

Choosing the right type to suit you can have enormous benefits for your health, so it's worth spending some time with your pendulum to help you make the right choices for you rather than being persuaded by others to do something you hate.

Crystal healing

Dowsing and crystal healing work together extremely well.

As a crystal healer, I prefer to work with a crystal dowsing pendulum and I do find that the crystal pendulum will be more in tune with other healing crystals, but you don't have to limit yourself to that, you can still work with a wooden or brass dowsing pendulum if you prefer, whichever you feel most comfortable with.

When you work with healing crystals, you are working with the healing energy of natural gemstones, the crystalline forms of minerals, that are provided for us by Mother Earth.

You are not working with the man-made, glass stones that are often called crystals when they are used for jewellery or for home decor.

Although crystal healing is a huge subject and one that I have written a number of detailed books about, the basis of crystal healing is very simple to work with.

Each different type of crystal or mineral has different energy, a different electromagnetic field and will interact with different parts of your own magnetic field.

There are dozens of different minerals and healing crystals available easily in gift shops, and hundreds available from specialist suppliers, either in some of the wonderful little shops that stock various types of alternative therapy such as aromatherapy, healing crystals, herbal remedies, Bach flower remedies and homeopathy, or from those who specialise in healing crystals and minerals.

If you have trouble finding one of these magical places locally, you can also find a very good supply of healing crystals on the Internet.

You can work with healing crystals in all areas of your life to help ease physical problems and to balance emotional, spiritual and mental energies.

You can also work with healing crystals to improve the atmosphere of your home or work environment, they can help you sleep, they can help you absorb information as you are studying, they can help protect you from low level electro-magnetic fields and the negative energy of other people around you.

The crystals that we use for their healing energy are the crystalline forms of minerals and most of them are beautiful.

You will be familiar with many of them from the world of jewellery.

Citrine, amethyst, rock crystal or clear quartz, sapphire, emerald, tourmaline, tigers eye, rose quartz, peridot, garnet and aquamarine - the list is almost endless.

All of these gemstones and many more, have different healing energies that can help balance your energy field and help to heal you.

They work on different layers of our energy field, the spiritual, the emotional, the mental and the physical.

You can work with single crystals or with many at the same time. You can set aside time to create healing layouts or you can simply wear or carry them with you every day.

Healing crystals can be used by anyone in almost any situation. You can even work with healing crystals to help your pets and animals. I work with rose quartz to help rescue animals regain their confidence and trust of humans.

Although the idea of working with crystals for their healing properties may sound strange, in fact we work with the energy of crystals every day without even thinking about it. The quartz movement in your watch is a paper thin piece of quartz which vibrates in response to an electric charge from the battery and allows the watch to keep good time and the transformation of quartz crystals into silicone chips has created the modern world.

Working with healing crystals.

When you want to work with the energy of a particular crystal or crystals you simply need to have it close to you, inside your electromagnetic field. You can visualise your energy field as a cocoon surrounding you at about arm's-length.

This means that you can carry your crystals in a pocket, place them on a desk in front of you as you work, I have many crystals around my computer as I write this.

You can also place them in a seat that you sit in regularly, hold them as you sit and relax or put them under your pillow as you sleep.

You can also wear them as jewellery of course and this is one of the easiest ways of keeping your crystals close to you on a regular basis.

You can work with many different crystals at the same time. Indeed, if you are working with a crystal layout you will be surrounded by many different energies working together to help balance your own energy field.

But what crystals should you use?

This is where your dowsing pendulum can help you.

You can dowse to help you choose the type of crystal you should work with for a particular problem or even which actual piece you should choose.

If you are buying your crystals from a specialist shop they won't have any problem with the idea of you working with your dowsing pendulum as you make your choices, dowsing over each different dish of crystals or over the individual pieces of amethyst or carnelian to find the one that you should choose for your own.

If you are at home and trying to narrow down your choices, you can create a set of cards for your healing crystals. You don't need to make a card for every type of crystal in your healing encyclopaedia, many of them will be very rare and difficult to get, and not the pieces you would begin your journey into crystal healing with.

Take some time to make your set of cards, it's worth spending time of creating this set of cards as you will use them again and again. You can add to your card set as time goes on and you become more experienced with your crystals. Although I have been working with healing crystals for over 20 years, I still dowse to check if a crystal is right for me or to work out which ones to use in new situations.

When you are working with your dowsing pendulum to discover which crystals you should work with, it's important to be clear in your mind about what exactly your question is.

Are you looking for crystals to help with a particular problem? Is it an intense but short term problem - a headache, a pulled muscle, a broken bone? Or is it a longer term or chronic problem, s serious injury or illness? Is it a physical problem or a problem caused by other people leading to stress and mental or emotional problems?

Once you have clarified your question and the purpose for which you want these crystals, you can start your dowsing session.

As always, you should begin your session by asking your pendulum if it is the right time to ask these questions.

As long as you receive the 'yes' response from your pendulum you can continue your session.

If you have created a set of cards, begin to dowse over each card in turn, focusing on your question and the reason you want to work with the crystal at this time.

You will probably receive a number of different 'yes' responses of different strengths and you may want to work with more than one crystal to balance your energy, as they can work on a single problem from different directions.

As well as choosing the type of crystal you should choose - amethyst, carnelian or charoite - you can also dowse to check what form you should choose. A polished piece set in jewellery, a large unpolished natural piece, a small tumbled stone or a carving?

You can also dowse to check that a specific piece is the right one for you. If I am choosing a new piece o jewellery I will work with my pendulum to make sure that it has good, positive energy and is a good crystal for me to wear.

Working with healing crystals is a constant matter of making choices and selecting which energies to work with, and much of it will become instinctive and natural as you become more used to the different energies, but there will still be times when you need a little more guidance and working with your pendulum will be a natural part of your crystal healing process.

You can also work with your dowsing pendulum to keep the energy of your crystals balanced.

As you work with healing crystal they absorb negative energy and this has to be cleansed from the crystal to keep it balanced.

There are many different ways of cleansing your crystals, some involve salt, some water and others the energy of the sun or moon, or the cleansing energy of a bed of amethyst, but I normally work with my pendulum to cleanse and balance the crystals I have been working with.

This is the same type of energy dowsing that you use when you are working to balance the chakras.

Ask your pendulum to balance the energy of the crystal and hold it over the piece.

Allow the pendulum to move as it wants to, and allow it to continue until it returns to the neutral or rest position, which will show that the energy has been balanced.

You should cleanse any crystal when you first receive it and then on a regular basis as you feel it needs recharging so that it can keep on working to balance your own energy field.

Energy cleansing

Energy is all around us.

Everything produces energy and it interacts with our own personal energy field.

The chapter on the chakra's deals with keeping your personal energy system in balance, but in this chapter I'm going to concentrate on how to understand the energy that surrounds you.

Some types of energy are positive, they recharge you, help you fill your own personal energy field with clear, clean energy that will help keep you healthy, happy and in balance with the universe.

Other types of energy will do the opposite. They will sap your own energy leaving you feeling tired, drained, depressed and can lead to depression, general unhappiness, disappointment and illness, even very serious illnesses.

The problem is that it's not always easy to see this negative energy and you can get so used to it, that you don't even feel it anymore, but it still has a negative effect on you.

It's easy to see an electricity pylon or substation, or a large factory or power station at the end of your garden. But it's not so easy to see underground power lines, an underground stream or lay lines.

All sorts of things can create an unhealthy energy area in your home and if you know what or where the problem is you can take action to eliminate, or at least minimise the effect.

You might even find that it is a person or group of people that are causing the problem and often it isn't the obvious culprit. Some people who are actually the cause of the trouble and bad atmosphere, are very good at hiding their true nature and causing other people to create the unrest while they play the part of peacemaker.

Some energies are in the environment and therefore difficult to avoid, but you can still protect yourself from them by introducing Feng Shui cures, being aware of them and using aromatherapy or crystals to protect yourself, and making sure that you balance your own personal energy frequently and recharge yourself with strong, clean, positive energy as often as possible.

Obviously you have to know that the negative energy is there in the first place, and your pendulum can help you tune into the energy that surrounds you, showing you whether it is negative or positive and how it will affect you personally.

Some negative energy is simply there, in the environment of a place, while we introduce a lot of it ourselves with our modern technology and some people are much more sensitive the low level electromagnetic fields that we surround ourselves with than others and will be much more aware of the discomfort that they can cause.

When you are dowsing for energy, you are asking your pendulum to show you if the energy is negative or positive.

Just hold the chain or cord of your pendulum gently so that you don't drop it and ask it to show you whether the energy is positive or negative. Your pendulum will give you it's 'yes', 'no' or neutral indicator and the size of the movement will let you see how weak or strong the energy field is. You will probably have to repeat this a number of times, moving across the area you are asking about. Some energy areas can be quite narrowly defined while others can cover a large area.

If you find areas of negative energy, you can either avoid them if you can, or work on ways to minimise their effect on you. You can ask a series of questions to find the most effective way of doing this.

- Should you use Feng Shui cures?
- Should you alter the use of the space?
- Should you wear personal crystal jewellery?
- Should you introduce healing crystals to the area?
- Should you use aromatherapy?
- Should you cleanse the space with smudging?

There are many different ways of balancing an area, and with some negative energies the best you can do is protect your own personal energy field from the worst of the negative effects. The questions you ask and the types of therapies and cures that you might want ask about, will vary with your individual circumstances and you should always use your own intuition when preparing your questions.

Unless you are lucky - and sensible - enough to spend all your time in areas of lovely, recharging, positive energy, you should also search out your own sanctuary of positive energy. Find a place that is close enough to where you live and work, where the energy is calming, peaceful and positive. It might be a park, the countryside if you are close enough to access it on a regular basic, a beautiful beach or coastal walk, a nature reserve or your own home or garden.

Once you have worked with your dowsing pendulum to find your personal oasis you should spend time in this pocket of positive energy as often as you can, especially of you spend other time in an area of negative energy and need to recharge yourself.

You can simply relax and absorb the positive atmosphere or you could meditate or do yoga, taking time to rebalance your own energy and protect yourself from the damaging effects of negative energy. Modern life seems have to developed the idea that spending time on yourself is self-indulgent, but if you don't look after your own energy and therefore your own health, you will be unable to look after anyone else or to be able to work effectively. Keeping your own energy balanced and positive is central to good health and wellbeing

As well as the natural energies of the Earth, we also surround ourselves with electrical equipment nowadays, from the computer that's sitting on my lap as I type at the moment (I use different computers as I work in different places!), to the TV's, mobile phones, fitness trackers, iPods and everything else that is wi-fi, Bluetooth and connected in the modern world. We live in a world of endless connections and we are constantly bombarded by radiation.

If you are thinking of buying a new piece of equipment, work with your dowsing pendulum to check that it will be good for you. After all, there's not much point in investing in the latest fitness tracker if the energy it produces is harming your health.

Once you have decided on the piece of equipment that you are interested in - but before you actually purchase it - work with your pendulum to find out if you should have that type of technology and what particular brand and model you should choose.

Make a list of all the varieties you could choose from. You can start by dowsing to find out which brand or type of equipment you should work with and, once you narrow it down, you can then dowse to find out which model in that range that would be best for you.

This is a very useful technique, because it is an area of life where there is a huge amount of pressure on your decision making. Advertising, social media pressure and peer pressure or even just the drive to have the latest piece of tech, all push you to different items, but this doesn't tell you anything about whether it will actually be good for you.

When you are dowsing about new electronic equipment, you shouldn't do it when you feel you just 'must have' the newest toy. Try to control the impulse to reach for the credit card and allow yourself some time to calm your mind.

Once you feel calm and relaxed, ask your pendulum if you can ask your questions. As long as you receive the 'yes' indicator, you can continue with your session.

As always, you must keep your emotions out of the dowsing session, try to forget how cool the latest, fanciest design is. The advertising, colour or list of extras don't actually make it the best item for you.

What you need to know is which piece of equipment will help rather than hinder your health, and that might mean that you should choose a more basic model. Of course, your pendulum might also show you that you shouldn't have that type of technology at all. Just because you want something doesn't mean it is good for you, and that is true in all areas of life.

Dowsing the home.

If you are in the process of choosing a new home, you should definitely spend some time with your pendulum to make sure that you pick a home whose energy will be helpful for you and your family. Ideally you will be able to find an oasis of positive energy that will feed you on every level, making life calmer, more successful and healthier, but at the very least you should avoid a place with damaging, negative energy.

Some houses or apartments have a very high turnover of residents and unfortunately seem to see a high number of serious illnesses or relationship break ups. You certainly don't want to move into that kind of energy blackspot, no matter how much pressure there is from the selling points of a good price, convenient schools or perfect interior.

You can either dowse over the address or property particulars or in the property itself, to check that the energy signature is positive and compatible for you and your family.

It's important to remain neutral as you do this dowsing.

You might be strongly drawn for property because of practical, 'logical' reasons.

It looks exactly right, it's in the right place, the price is lower than others you been looking at, or you're being pressurised by the agent who is telling you that other buyers are interested, have even made an offer.

But none of that will be of any consolation if you discover six months later that your happy family life has disintegrated into an endless stream of arguments and ill-health.

Calm your mind and focus totally on dowsing the energy of the property. As a dowsing session, this one is fairly straightforward. There are really only three answers.

It's either positive or negative energy or possibly negative that can be fixed by making alterations or adding some feng shui cures. For instance, it might need rewiring or changes to the plumbing. You might need to change the use of some of the rooms around or remove a large, overpowering and possibly damaged tree that is damaging the energy.

One thing you should also keep firmly in mind as you ask these questions, is a timeframe.

Is this a forever home or place for the next few years while you study?

Is it a main home or holiday home?

If you are looking at a property for the long-term, your forever home, it is probably worth making large alterations, such as having the property entirely rewired or adding an extension to add the feng shui area that it missing from the ground plan of the building.

The wealth area is in the far back left corner of the building when the outline of your home is looked at from the front door, while the relationship area is in the far right hand corner. The feng shui plan is easy to work out and there are cures that can compensate for a missing area. Some are very simple and easy to add, but if you are looking for a property for just the next year or two, it almost certainly isn't worth making a large of financial investment to alter the house - unless you are looking at it as an investment and developing the property to make a profit.

Once you have decided what type of property you're are actually looking for and what your purpose is, you can proceed with your dowsing session.

In general, almost any level of 'no' means you should reject that property, because your question should have included your purchasing purpose.

With the 'yes' response, obviously the stronger the indicator the better. If you receive a 'no - but' or 'yes - but' you should continue and ask further questions such as;

Would it need alterations and would these alterations be structural or just cosmetic?

Will the alterations be financially worthwhile?

How much time would it take? A month, 18 months?

And of course would be investment in time and money, make the energy of the property right for you?

Of course most of us are already in a home and want to make the energy in that home, work as well as it can.

Again you need to approach this as calmly as possible.

You have to be able to detach yourself from the emotional baggage that is normally involved when there are problems in the home.

You should try and avoid taking out your dowsing pendulum at the end of another serious row, while you are dealing with an illness - either yourself or a with a member of your family - or when you are feeling depressed and despondent.

If the problems are serious, try and remove yourself from the home altogether and do your dowsing session in a place of safe, positive energy.

Most of us don't have the freedom to simply move, although you may find that you should make that a priority rather than a distant dream.

You can ask if the energy of your home can be improved - most can be.

Should you alter the use of the rooms? Turn a bedroom into an office and vice-versa or move the office out of the home altogether?

Should you change some of the equipment? Is the microwave oven causing a negative energy flow or should the cordless phone be taken out of the bedroom?

- Should you redecorate with different colours?
- Should you add feng shui cures?
- Should you add crystal healing cures?
- Should you smudge to cleanse the space, purifying the area with the smoke of sacred herbs such as sage, cedar or lavender?
- Should you declutter? Clutter can stop the flow of energy.
- Should you work with aromatherapy to freshen the energy?
- Should you move the furniture around?
- Does the whole house have to be tackled or is a single room causing the problems?
- Should you redesign the garden?

There are almost as many questions are there are people and homes, because all of us are individuals and groups of individual families, and we all have our own needs, so think about the problems you want to deal with and prepare your questions for your dowsing session.

Of course you don't have to be experiencing serious problems, almost all of us can improve the energy of the home we live in, tweaking small things and making small cures to move it closer to perfect.

Dealing with pain.

Your dowsing pendulum can be a wonderful tool for unwinding pain.

Pain can come from all sorts of causes.

You can have painful feet after standing too long or walking around too many shops in uncomfortable shoes.

You can have a headache after too many hours sitting in front of the computer or listening to loud voices.

You can have back pain from an uncomfortable seating position or from twisting as you work.

So many of the normal everyday things we do can cause aches and pains, just take a look at how many boxes of painkillers can be found on supermarket shelves.

So next time you have aches and pains, reach for your dowsing pendulum rather than the box of pills.

When you are dowsing to relieve pain you will be using a different technique than when doing most dowsing.

Rather than asking a question or series of questions to get a 'yes' or 'no', a negative or positive response, for pain relief you will be working with your pendulum in the same method as you do for energy balancing - in fact you are balancing the energy to ease the pain.

You start this process in the same way as more traditional dowsing.

Ask your pendulum if you can work with it to relieve the pain.

As always, be very specific in your question. You need to be accurate in exactly what pain you want to relieve.

If your pendulum indicates 'yes', you can continue but if it indicates 'no' or 'yes - but' you should ask more questions before going any further.

If the indicator is 'yes - but', ask if you can relieve the pain now but then consult a doctor about the cause. If the answer to that is 'yes' you can focus in on the timeframe. Should you consult the doctor within the month, the week, tomorrow?

These are some other suggestions for the type of question might want ask.

Should I get a medical opinion in the near future?

Should I learn how to make changes in my life to avoid a repetition of the pain? Sometimes if you just keep relieving pain or ache, you don't tackle the actual cause of it, and the underlying problem can get worse.

If the indicator is 'no', again you can ask further questions to find out why your pendulum is giving you a 'no' response.

An important question to ask in this case is, should I go to the hospital now? You will normally receive a 'no' indicator to this question, but better sure than sorry.

Most of the time when asking if you can continue with your dowsing to unwind pain, your indicator will be 'yes' and you can continue with your dowsing session to relieve that pain.

You can either hold the pendulum over the painful area, or you can hold your free hand over the pain and dowse with the other hand in a more comfortable position. You'll quickly cause other aches if you try to hold your pendulum over your head to ease a headache!

You can also simply focus your attention on the pain that you want to ease while you are dowsing.

Sit comfortably and don't cross your legs, you don't want to enclose or trap the energy.

Ask your pendulum to relieve or ease the pain that you want to work on, and just allow your pendulum to move as it wants to, for as long as it wants, until it comes back to its neutral position.

There are no hard and fast rules about how long this will take, a few seconds or a few minutes.

I find that I can tell the different types of pain when I am dowsing a client.

If the pain is severe but temporary, for instance headache from too much noise, a sore throat from being in a long meeting, an insect sting or blisters from walking or back ache from too many hours at the computer, the pendulum will move in large patterns but will come back to neutral fairly quickly, normally within about 60 to 90 seconds. This indicates that, although the pain may be severe, it is not serious and once eased the effects should last for quite a while or relieve the problem altogether until you repeat the thing that caused it in the first place.

However, if the pendulum continues to move for three or four minutes, even though the movement is smaller, this normally indicates that the pain is more deeply rooted in the energy field.

Sometimes the cause is well known, one of my clients suffers back pain from falling from a horse a number of years ago. A series of dowsing sessions over 3 to 4 days can help ease the pain for a number of months, but it will return and the pendulum always takes a while to balance the pain in the first session, getting quicker over the days.

At other times you may not know the cause of the pain and in this case you should consult a doctor or, if you are dowsing someone else, you should suggest that they consult their doctor.

It is extremely important to remember that pain has a purpose.

It is there to warn you about a problem. It is a signal that something is wrong and you should never ignore constant or regular pain. If the pain lasts, you need to take notice of it and get professional medical advice.

Do not just keep getting rid of the pain, whether by taking tablets or by dowsing. Find out why it hurts.

If you do take medical advice and find that no treatment is needed or available, and that you just have to live with the pain, by all means go ahead and work with your pendulum for pain relief.

Dowsing doesn't come with side effects!

As long as you know that the pain isn't an indicator of a more serious problem, you can dowse to relieve the pain as often as you like.

If you discover that it is the symptom of a more serious illness, you can continue to work with your pendulum to balance your energy field but you should not use it as a replacement for medical treatment you should use it to compliment the treatment.

Emotional healing

Emotional, mental or spiritual stress can be one of the main causes for many illnesses and for general lack of health.

If you are under emotional pressure and stress it can lead to all sorts of problems.

Physically it can mean that you don't look after yourself properly, you may not eat healthily, you might not feel like exercising, you might not feel like engaging with friends, you may drink too much alcohol, smoke too many cigarettes and cause all sorts of other problems that will cause physical health problems in the short or long term.

But it is more than that.

Stress can eat into your energy field.

Dealing with the stress of a broken relationship, or bereavement. Dealing with a difficult employment situation, dealing with family or financial problems or even being seriously unhappy with your living conditions, can wear you down. It can eat into your energy field, your chakras and cause physical illnesses.

Even Western medicine now accepts that stress can weaken your immune system, making you more likely to suffer from infections and even more susceptible to chronic illnesses such as high blood pressure, diabetes, IBS, and even cancer.

All of this means that, far from putting up with stress, it is definitely something to deal with and in many cases eradicate.

There are certain levels of stresses that are actually healthy, some people do not react well to living a very quiet, balanced, and stress-free life. They thrive on challenges and a regular burst of adrenaline. Within reason there is nothing wrong with this, although if taken to extremes, adrenaline can be addictive and damaging to the body.

But as a general guide, the stress, excitement and adrenaline rush of rock climbing, skydiving, water-skiing or snowboarding is not something to worry about.

The adrenaline rush of a high-powered career, constantly making decisions and dealing daily with solving problems and creating solutions, this can be very empowering and very exciting.

The problem comes when the stress is too much, the emotional damage is too draining, and the mental exhaustion becomes unbearable. The kind of stress where you are not in control.

Dowsing can help you untangle the knots that uncontrolled stress can cause in life.

When you are in the midst of an extremely stressful situation, it can be impossible to see anything outside or beyond your immediate situation, and that can mean that you are unable to see the answers or even the true cause of distress.

Although it might seem virtually impossible, find a calm corner in your life for your dowsing session.

Find a place and time where you won't be disturbed. Turn your phone and emails off, the world can manage without you for a while.

Play some relaxing music or light some scented candles if it helps you to relax. You could have a cup of chamomile tea or use an aromatherapy diffuser, just use something that works for you, although remember that alcohol - and that includes wine - is actually a depressant and a sedative that affects the central nervous system, so you shouldn't learn to rely on it to relax you after a long day, as it can make your levels of anxiety worse over time.

Sit comfortably with your back straight.

Breathe in slowly through your nose, filling the whole of your lungs, counting slowly from one to five, although you shouldn't force it and you might have to work up to the count of five.

Let the breath escaped slowly through your mouth, again counting slowly to five.

Breathe without pausing or holding your breath, and notice that I have said 'slowly' a number of times. It's called slow breathing for a reason.

Ideally you should do this for a few minutes - between three and five - until you feel relaxed and calm.

This is also a technique you can use in general, throughout the day to help calm your stress levels.

Once you have calmed your mind, you can begin your dowsing session.

First of all, you should ask your pendulum if you can begin your session.

If you receive the 'no' indicator it might be the wrong time. You might still be too stressed or not emotionally detached enough, come back to it at another time, but don't leave it too long.

As long as you have prepared and calmed yourself you should receive the 'yes' indicator and you can continue your session.

You should have prepared your questions in advance. Clarity in your questions is one of the most important parts of dowsing and it can be difficult to hold that clarity when you are general suffering the problems caused by stress.

Your pendulum can give you 'yes' and 'no', even 'yes - but' and 'no - but'. It can even give you 'unanswerable' and 'stupid question' indicators if you take the time to do advanced programing with your pendulum in the first place, but you still have to begin with a clear question if you want to be able to get a meaningful answer.

Preparing these questions be quite difficult and the range of questions will vary depending on what areas of your life are causing you to feel so tense and unwell.

It might be that you are not even sure what area is causing the problem. After all problems at work can cause you to be irritable and uncommunicative at home which will cause stress in your relationship.

Problems with a child can cause you to be distracted at work and lead to a fresh set of problems with your boss.

Being bullied by someone can lead to the type of stress and depression that can leak out into all parts of your life.

Turning the tap off on the cause is the only way to improve all the other problems.

You could have a succession of different jobs, but if the problem stems from a personal relationship, changing your job won't solve the problem.

Equally, a stress source in your career won't be solved by a string of unsuccessful, romantic relationships.

So the first question for your pendulum is to find the source of your problem.

- Is the source financial?
- Is the source your family?
- Is the source your general lifestyle?
- Is the source your career?
- Is the source your past?
- Is the source the people you call friends?
- Is the source your spiritual health?

Although these are some general starting places, the number of questions and possibilities probably match the number of people on the planet.

You are the only person who can work out your own questions and you will find that it will take you on your own personal journey. You just have to trust your intuition and the answers that you get from your dowsing pendulum as you start on your journey to relieving stress.

For some people the answer might be quite straightforward. You really are working in a place that is wrong for you and you have to move on, and no matter how difficult that seems to be, everything will fall into a much better place once you remove the source of the stress and negative energy in your life.

For most of us it will be a bit more complex and for some it might mean a complete change of career with retraining, a move across the country and a whole new life with new friends and new partner, before they find the life that they should be living.

But stress can destroy your life and if you are suffering from serious stress it is worth spending some time to find out why you are suffering so much stress and how you can make the difference to make life worthwhile and enjoyable.

Be prepared to spend time with your pendulum to work through the areas of your life that are causing the emotional pressure and stress.

It has probably taken a number of years to reach this stage and if you have reached the limits of your energy it is difficult to think clearly and to find the time to work on fixing the problems, but whatever stage you have reached, it is possible to rebalance your energy and work your way back to a calmer place.

Work with your pendulum to find out which type of alternative therapy will help you to deal with the stress. You might find that you need to introduce feng shui cures and aromatherapy into your home, healing crystals into your work place either as pieces in your pocket or on your desk or as jewellery. You might find that you need to make time for exercise or time in the open air, time to spend on yourself, going for shopping with friends or a regular facial, reiki session or back massage. Or you might find that you need to make the effort to learn new skills, re-train and work on creating the life you always really wanted rather than the logical choices that were made for you.

Ideally you will be dealing with balancing the stress before it gets too serious and will keep your energy field in balance. Stress hits everyone at some time, and for most of us it will happen on a regular basis at a low level. Recognising this and working with your pendulum to track the source and find solutions will help you healthy and happy.

Finding a practitioner

Although there are lots of ways in which you can improve your health and well-being through diet, exercise, home treatment and lifestyle changes, there are times when you will need to work with a particular practitioner.

This can be anything from choosing a regular therapist, a homeopath, a chiropractor, a new dentist or choosing which hospital you would prefer to go to for an operation.

The choices you make in these cases can have a profound effect on your health and you should never make them lightly.

You may want to choose between different types of practitioner.

For instance, back pain can be very difficult type of pain to trace to its source. It can be a physical problem such as skeletal or muscular, it can be caused by tension, poor posture, illness, incorrect exercise, injury or even by the wrong shoes or chair that you use.

Should you see a physiotherapist, a chiropractor, a Reiki therapist, an acupuncturist, a reflexologist, or go for an aromatherapy massage? Or should you go to your doctor and insist on further tests and possibly a scan.

Pain is the body's warning system and you should never ignore it or simply find ways of blocking it, either with over-the-counter painkillers, prescription drugs or alternative therapies.

Serious recurring pain is there for a reason. Find out what the reason is, otherwise the painkillers might turn out to be real killers.

Once you know the cause of the pain, it might be something that you have to learn to live with, and at that stage you can certainly find ways to live with it more comfortably and finding a practitioner might well be the way or one of the ways that you choose to do that.

First of all, you will need to decide which type of therapy that you will work with. Reiki or reflexology? Aromatherapy or acupuncture?

Either write a list of the different types of practitioner or create a set of dowsing cards with each type of practitioner or treatment written on a separate card.

Prepare for your dowsing session.

Don't simply reach for your pendulum when you are in pain, the emotional effect will interfere with accurate dowsing.

Find a calm place where you will not be disturbed. Turn off your phone and emails and create a haven of calm for yourself. Play relaxing music, light scented candles or use aromatherapy if that helps you to relax. Make sure that you wear comfortable clothing.

Focus on the reason you are looking for a practitioner. Are you looking for yourself, your partner, a parent or child?

You must focus your thoughts, otherwise you might think that you are asking for yourself but actually be thinking about how bad your mother's arthritis has been this week, and that would confuse your dowsing session.

Concentrate on exactly what health issues you want to deal with and what timescale you are looking for. Do you want treatment for an immediate injury or a therapist to help with a long term chronic illness?

Ask your pendulum if you can proceed with this dowsing session at this time.

You will normally receive the 'yes' indicator for this. If you receive the 'no' indicator you can just put your pendulum away until another time or you could ask further questions to find out why you received the 'no' indicator. Are you too stressed, upset or emotionally involved at the moment? That would have to be three separate questions.

Are you waiting for test results? You may need to wait until you receive them before deciding on any therapy or treatment.

As long as you receive the 'yes' indicator you can proceed with your session.

First you need to narrow down the list of therapies. Your pendulum might indicate a single therapy or a combination or two or more.

You will also need to ask further questions to decide which therapies and treatments you might work with in the longer term, what time periods should be involved and whether the therapies should be used together or as a journey through your healing.

For instance, your dowsing may indicate that you should start with a short intense session of physiotherapy followed by an exercise plan for you to continue at home and then supported by aromatherapy massage on a regular basis.

Every situation is different, which means that every set of questions and answers will also be different and unique to you.

Once you have narrowed down the type of therapy that you should choose, you also need to make a choice of exactly which therapist or clinic you should go to!

You can compose your list from information available locally in local papers, in magazines, professional directories as well as from Internet and of course the best way is if you can receive a personal recommendation from a friend - although in this case you should still dowse to ensure that the therapist will be the right choice for you. The fact that someone was perfect for your friend does not mean that their energy will be a suitable match for your own.

If you have decided that you need to make more regular visits you probably want to limit the distance you would travel.

Again this is a matter of personal preference. While 10 miles can be a long journey for some people, 100 miles will be a daily commute for others.

And of course, if you are looking for a specialist that you might only visit once, or for an initial treatment for a week or two, you might decide that a trip to a different country is a worthwhile investment in time and money.

Once you have decided on the possible therapists, you can create a set of dowsing cards.

Unlike a set of dowsing cards for Bach flower remedies or aromatherapy, that you will keep and use for many different sessions, this set will probably be only used the once to help you find the therapist you want to work with for this problem.

The person you are looking for not only has to be good at their therapy, it's very important that you are comfortable with their style, their methods and their energy. A friend of mine likes very deep tissue massage, where as it just hurts me and does more harm than good, so although we go to the same clinic we prefer different therapists.

You can create this set of cards on paper rather than card. Cut a sheet into regular sized pieces and write each therapists name or clinic on a separate piece. If you choose a clinic first, then you should continue your dowsing to choose the individual therapist.

Lay out the pieces on a clear table with space between each piece. The table should be clear so that nothing else on it will affect your dowsing. For instance, if you have a bowl decorated with lotus flowers and one of the clinics has lotus in their name, the result could be influenced subconsciously.

Sit comfortably and calm yourself with some deep slow breaths.

Keep the purpose of your question clearly in mind and dowse over each card asking your pendulum to show you if this is the therapist that you are looking for.

As you are now looking for a therapist in a single discipline you will normally only find a single 'yes'.

If the pendulum gives you more than one 'yes' indicator and you will have to ask more questions to make your final choice. Does one involve more travelling? Is there a large difference in cost? Does one of them offer other therapies that would also suit you?

Take time to think about the information you have gathered so far and to clarify your thoughts so that you can ask other questions. You might want to take a rest to clear your mind before continuing possibly for a few minutes, a few hours or even a few days. It is important to get the right answer not quick answer.

Conclusion

I hope that this has given you a taste of the ways in which you can work with your dowsing pendulum to help improve your health and wellbeing and that it has shown you the different paths that you can take to a healthier lifestyle.

There are many types of alternative therapy and complimentary medicine that you can choose from, and many can be combined to create a positive and nourishing energy in your home, your family and your own personal space, and dowsing can help you find the ones that are right for you.

The longer you work with your dowsing the more comfortable you will feel and the more natural it will become, helping you focus your thought, tune into your subconscious and helping you hear the wisdom of the energies that surround us.

I hope that you enjoy the journey.

About the Author

From a long line of healers on the West Coast of Ireland, Brenda has worked with a dowsing pendulum and healing crystals for over 15 years and is a member of the British Society of Dowsers.

She regularly gives talks and classes on dowsing, vibrational therapies, crystal healing and colour healing as well as writing books, articles and well known series of Core Information charts on a number of alternative therapies.

you can contact her at:

brenda@healing-earth.co.uk

website: www.healing-earth.co.uk

Also by Brenda Hunt

A Beginner's Guide to Pendulum Dowsing
Dowsing and the Chakra System
Dowsing for a happy, healthy home
Dowsing and your garden

A Beginner's Guide to the Chakra System
A Beginner's Guide to working with healing crystals

Healing crystals - a guide to working with series

A guide to working with Amethyst
A guide to working with Rose Quartz
A guide to working with Obsidian
A guide to working with Carnelian
A guide to working with Citrine
A guide to working with Tourmaline